Shaolin Temple

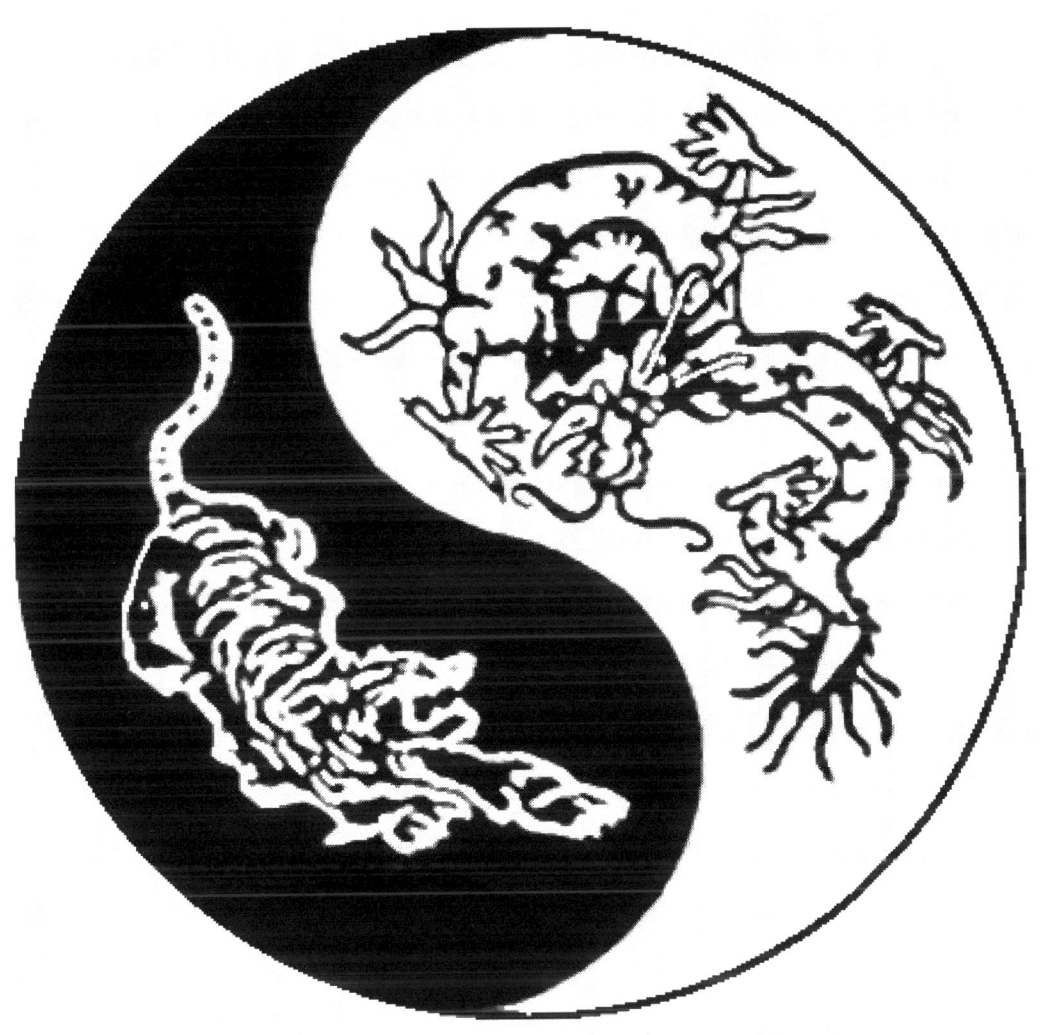

Monk Manual
and
Esoteric Teachings

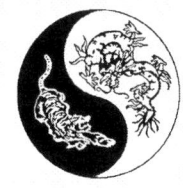

Shaolin Temple: Monk Manual and Esoteric Teachings

Copyright © 2010 by Thomas F. Smith

ISBN: 9781079544541

All rights are reserved, including the right of reproduction, in whole or in part, in any form.

Published by the Shaolin Temple,
Educational and Literature Department
6345 Newburgh, Westland, Michigan
48185

Printed and manufactured in the
United States of America

DISCLAIMER
 The Shaolin Temple, author(s) and publisher of this material are **not responsible** in any manner whatsoever for any injury which may occur through reading or following the instructions in this material.
 Some of the activities described in this material may be too strenuous for some people.
A medical examination and consultation with a doctor may be required before engaging in them.

I salute the Supreme Teacher, the Truth,

whose nature is Bliss;

who is the giver of the highest happiness;

who is pure Wisdom;

who is beyond all qualities and infinite like the sky;

who is beyond words;

who is one and eternal, pure and still;

who is beyond all change and phenomena

and who is the silent witness to all our thoughts and emotions-

I salute Truth, the Supreme Teacher.

-Ancient Vedic Hymn

DEDICATION:

To my wife Janine,
whose dedication to Truth
has enabled the writing of this book.

To the saints, sages and monks,
whose spiritual awareness and compassion
have made this knowledge and Wisdom available to us.

And to all the seekers
that will use these sacred teachings
to assist in the positive evolution of themselves and Humanity.

TABLE OF CONTENTS

Introduction xiv

Part I
Orientation

Shaolin Tradition...1 - 1
Timeline of Philosophical Influences...1 - 2
Bodhidarma Background..1 - 4
Bodhidarma Stories..1 - 7
Kshatriya Ethics and Influence...1 - 11
Areas of Self Development..1 - 12
Aspects of Spirit..1 - 12
Aspects of Physical Fitness...1 - 12
Aspects of Health..1 - 12
Leaders; Master Sensei Eizo Onishi ....1 - 13
Comments on Discipline; Lord Shiva...1 - 13
Water Metaphor of Spirit; Yogacharya, Sri John Oliver Black........................1 - 14
Comparison of Moral Codes and Discipline...1 - 15
Genealogy (Chart)...1 - 16
Historical Map..1 - 17
Influence of the Original Five Animal Methods of the Shaolin Tradition........1 - 18

The Spirit Warrior..1 - 21
    Difference between a Warrior and a Soldier...1 - 21
    The 1st and 2nd Task; The Spirit Warrior becomes a Bodhisattva............1 - 21
    Responsibility for the Self..1 - 22
    Self Examination / Personality Purification - The Battlefield of the Spirit Warrior ..1 - 23
    The Worldly Paradigm; Spiritual Ignorance..1 - 24
    Detachment...1 - 25
    Truth, Will ....1 - 26
    Optimism and Gratitude..1 - 27
    Forgiveness of Others and the Self..1 - 27
    Self Mastery..1 - 28
    Will...1 - 29
    Complete Spiritual Realization Is Inevitable..1 - 31

The Summary of the Monk's Orientation
    The Monk's Vow..1 - 32

Table of Contents (continued)

Part II
Goals and Methods

Goals and Methods of the Shaolin Tradition..2 - 1
Learning Methods   Self Examination\Personality Purification..................2 - 2
                               Energization of Consciousness...............................2 - 2
                               The Five Perfections..2 - 3
                               Positive Change / Self Discovery Learning..............2 - 4
                               The Warning...2 - 4
                               Spiritual Ignorance..2 - 5
                               Intellectual Limitations..2 - 6
Learning Methods Used   Meditation..2 - 8
   in the Shaolin Tradition   Hsing (forms)...2 - 9
                               Chi Kung...2 - 10
                               Technique Drills..2 - 10
                               Partner Practice...2 - 10
                               San Shou..2 - 11
                               The Detriment of Competition...............................2 - 11
General Direction for Study - Advice from Onishi Sensei.................................2 - 12

Part III
Meditation

Meditation: Concentration Used to Know God............................3 - 1
   What it is   Four Stages of Meditation.......................................3 - 3
     Why it is done   Suggestions for Meditation.....................................3 - 4
       How to do it   Mantra Use...3 - 4
                                 Meditation Instructions..3 - 5
Meditation   Anuloma Viloma...3 - 6
   Preparation   Bandas...3 - 7
    Techniques   Head Drop..3 - 7
                                 Maha Mudra...3 - 8
                                 Uddiyana Pranayama..3 - 10
                                 Supta-Vajrasan..3 - 11
Sense Withdrawal   Wu Hsin...3 - 12
    Techniques   Yoni Mudra..3 - 13
                                 Jesus on the Light of God......................................3 - 14
Satori Techniques   Soo Hum Meditation Technique..............................3 - 15
                                 Omm Meditation..3 - 16
                                 Chakra Light Meditation..3 - 17
Krishna on Meditation: The Song Celestial...3 - 18

xi
Table of Contents (continued)

Part IV
Training Methods for Spiritual Chi Kung

Chi Kung

  Chi Introduction..4 - 1

Background Info for Spiritual Chi Kung

  Five Primary Training Methods..4 - 3
  Chakra Developmental Maturity Construct..4 - 4
  Spiritual Birth, Origin of the Bridal Chamber Sacrament...................4 - 8
  Chakra Correlation within the Lord's Prayer......................................4 - 11

Preparatory Exercises

  Sea Salt Detoxification..4 - 14
  Fasting...4 - 15
  Stretching and Routines..4 - 16
  Energization Exercise and Yoga Nidra...4 - 18

Consciousness Energization Exercises (Spiritual Chi Kung)

  Energy Loss Due to Stress ....4 - 19
  Breathing ....4 - 20
  Crane Breath...4 - 21
  Chart of Primary Vessels for Chi Transportation...............................4 - 22

Classic Hsing (Forms) as Spiritual Chi Kung

  The Mystical Meaning of the Mudra and Movements of San Zan.............4 - 23
  San Zan and Chi Kung and Guidelines for Practice...................................4 - 29
  The Affirmations for the Practice of San Zan..4 - 30
  Sei San Chuan Diagram and Performance Information.............................4 - 31
  San Sei Chuan Diagram and Performance Information.............................4 - 32
  The Mystical Meaning of the Mudra and Movements of Pai He Chuan...4 - 34

Summary Concepts of Chi Kung Training

  Principles of Chi Kung Practice..4 - 42
  Important Concepts in Chi Kung..4 - 43

Table of Contents (continued)

Part V
Training Methods for Martial Technique

Introduction		5 - 1
Temple Forms ----	Temple Hsing	5 - 2
	Classic Hsing	5 - 2
	Wu Hsin in Forms Training	5 - 4
Martial Technique -	Soft Versus Hard	5 - 6
	Stance, Posture	5 - 7
	Eye Position and Gaze	5 - 8
	Hand Position	5 - 8
	Technique Power	5 - 8
	Hand Techniques	5 - 9
	Kicking Techniques	5 - 9
	Fighting Strategies	5 - 10
	Mobility	5 - 11
	Training Tips	5 - 12
	Taolu Technique List	5 - 13
	List of Stepping Patterns	5 - 14
Martial Forms		5 - 15
	Wu Hsing Chuan Combination Sets	5 - 15
	Graph of Wu Hsing Chuan Combination Directions	5 - 16

Part VI
Requirements for Monastic Training

Application for Acceptance as a Shaolin Monk	6 - 1
Levels of Monastic Training	6 - 2
Required Reading List	6 - 2
Monks Vow	6 - 3
Purpose of Ceremony	6 - 4
Prayer and Prayers	6 - 5
Singing Bowl Ritual	6 - 8
Healing Ritual	6 - 9
Lunar and Solar Spiritual Eye Ritual	6 - 10
Chakra Energization Ritual	6 - 11
Annual Global Peace Ritual	6 - 12
Days of Commemoration	6 - 13
Mudra: Symbolism and Use	6 - 15
Mudra Lists	6 - 16

Table of Contents (continued)

Part VII
Monastic Initiation and Monastic Requirements

Grading and Evaluation
      General Grading Information..7 - 1
      Criteria for the Evaluation of Hsing...7 - 1
      Criteria for the Evaluation of Written Assignments...............................7 - 2

Monastic Requirements
      Student Monk Test Description..7 - 3
            Student Monk Testing Information...7 - 4
            Class Opening Ceremony..7 - 5
            Academic Reading Requirements Description..........................7 - 6
      Disciple Monk Test Description...7 - 7
            Academic Reading Requirements Description..........................7 - 8
      Monk Test Description..7 - 9
            Academic Reading Requirements Description..........................7 - 10
            Cobra Breath Warning...7 - 11
      Priest Test Description..7 - 12
            Academic Reading Requirements Description..........................7 - 13

Appendix

A Self Analysis Chart..A - 1
B Testing Initiation Application Forms...A - 2
C Monk Readiness - Self Assessment...A - 3
D Tao Chang Rules...A - 6

Bibliography - Suggested Reading List..B - 1

Glossary of Terms...C - 1

Instructional Aids Available...D - 1

INTRODUCTION TO THE SHAOLIN TEMPLE MONK MANUAL

The purpose of this text is to present the teachings of Shaolin Tradition. The practice of these teachings can culminate into the experience of merging the individual self with the Universal Self (the Great Spirit). This experience is required to solve the problem of stress and suffering and fill the experience of life with Joy. The Shaolin Tradition was developed to prepare people to efficiently interact within the worldly realm and to train them to disseminate the teachings to others that can appreciate and use them.

The worldly paradigm is the faulty orientation to life created by the individual self (ego) for the purpose of making sense out of reality and attempting to efficiently interact with it. The information the ego uses to develop this orientation is based on the experiences it can get from the five senses and the minds ability to assemble the information into a usable form. These senses evolved to interact with the earth environment and nothing more, they can not collect information beyond our universe. The problem is that the vast majority of Reality exits beyond our universe, inaccessible to the senses and the intellect. Through the intellect alone, the ego does not have the knowledge or experience to apprehend Reality. The belief system based on this orientation is the cause of all stress and suffering. The only way to solve this problem is through a personal intuitive experience of Spirit. This experience will not only free the individual self from all stress and suffering but it will also imbue ones consciousness with Spirit and all its aspects (e.g. Infinite Love, Light, Compassion, Truth, Wisdom, Joy, etc.).

Intuition is the ability of the awareness to apprehend a concept or experience without physical evidence (the use of the senses or intellect). A mystic is someone who realizes that intuition is the key to this experience of Spirit and the accurate apprehension of Reality. This, therefore, can be a manual for mystics, who want to solve the problem of stress and suffering and make this experience available to others.

Things the Mystic must know before one can efficiently begin.

The mystic must accept responsibility for the development of their own spiritual awareness. Some assistance can be obtained but the Five Perfections must be incorporated into the mystics personality first. Also the mystic must accept responsibility for all their own thoughts, behaviors and circumstances. Our *own* choices determine what happens in our lives.

Efficient intuitional ability depends on high levels of psychic energy (chi/prana). In the Shaolin Tradition, these energy levels are raised through the practice of consciousness energization exercises. These exercises include both physical and mental aspects (e.g. asanas, hsing (kata), physical movement, mudra, mantra, affirmations, visualizations, breath control, energy transportation and accumulation, meditation, etc.). It is these consciousness energization exercises which make the Shaolin Tradition a method of kundalini yoga.

Introduction (continued)

The experience of Spirit depends on the incorporation of the aspects of Spirit into the personality of the individual self (the ego). In fact, spiritual awareness is directly proportional to the incorporation of the aspects of Spirit into the personality. This is accomplished through the practice of the Shaolin personality purification methods and through the practice of meditation.

The mystic can expect that the sincere and disciplined practice of Shaolin Tradition will bring: greater physical health, the elimination stress and suffering, and a direct experience of Spirit and all its aspects.

The policy of the Shaolin Tradition in its approach to knowledge, is that one is **not** expected to believe anything just because an authority figure says it is so or because it is written in a revered book. All information is to be personally examined, tested and experienced before it is accepted as valid or usable; and examined, tested and experienced again when contradictory information is obtained.

In order to obtain satisfactory results, daily practice of both the consciousness energization exercises and the sitting meditation is required. To receive the benefits that the practice that the Shaolin Tradition can bring, it is highly recommended that the student set aside a few minutes each day to review and practice the movements and methods that are being trained and applied.

It has been said that the objectives of the Shaolin Tradition are harmony of the Mind, promotion of health, and the attainment of rejuvenation and longevity. Bodhidharma said that with the direct experience of Spirit, everything will become available: the end of stress and suffering, the facilitation of mental stability, excellent health, rejuvenation, longevity and the efficient ability to interact with Reality.

INTRODUCTION
By Kancho Eizo Onishi

Ken Do Gaku

The Chinese characters for "Ken" suggest martial art. "Do" simply means "road," used in the metaphorical way, and consists of a long, complex process of personal development. "Gaku" means "study" that is firmly based on logic and reason, not merely a compendium of individual styles – it may be said to be the object of Ken Do Gaku. Thus, "the study of the way of Ken", does not consist only of martial skills or an accepted system of beliefs, it encompasses a wide body of knowledge always growing and changing as more evidence is obtained.

The pursuit of Ken Do Gaku involves thinking without regard for one's likes or dislikes. When this thought process results in scientific, logical knowledge, the requirements suggested by the word "Gaku" are met. Because Ken Do Gaku is a "study", it is more than a limited competition for rank or sport, whose object is to win.

Ken Do Gaku is an unlimited field that can accommodate many interests or lines of research. New approaches and new areas for development are likewise unlimited. As an inquiry into the nature of Ken, Ken Do Gaku is a field of study in its own right, with distinctive research procedures and objectives. Therefore, Gaku (the study) is at least as important as the art because it is the means of obtaining achievement in the art.

Study Objectives

Throughout the ages, there have been men who have devoted their lives to the study of fighting techniques to answer the various needs of their particular historical periods. Ken Do Gaku strives to further this process of an going discovery for the benefit of the people and society of this age.

Further, Ken Do Gaku objectives are the fostering between the people of the world the spirit of believing in one another and helping each other, in living their lives enjoyably in peace and health. Founded on the spirit of love of humanity, Ken do Gaku, both from its cultural and martial aspects, aims to uncover the right ways for human beings to live their lives. This spirit applies to everyone, regardless of class, country, or race. It is a spirit of harmony that lends humanity to human relations.

Introduction (continued)

The Quality of Humanity

The image of man as often represented in popular culture contains little regarding his physiological or psychological makeup. Religion, on the other hand, often stresses his psychological aspects when its purpose should be the spiritual. Religion, in general, completely excludes any consideration of his physiological characteristics. Ken Do Gaku considers both aspects of man. It cultivates man's physical and inner being harmoniously, producing a well-rounded human being.

Instruction Policy

The concentration is on independent study, without relying on others. Answers are not given; answers must be scientifically valid. All knowledge must be self validated with direct experience before it is accepted as truth. Also Ken do Gaku is not merely theory; knowledge must be put into action.

Study

Ken Do gaku can be carried out only with an earnest attitude. It is not for people with treacherous intentions. It will not bring one worldly riches. It is a thing to be studied, a method of human growth.

Eizo Onishi
Founder of Koei Kan Ken Do Gaku

PART I

ORIENTATION

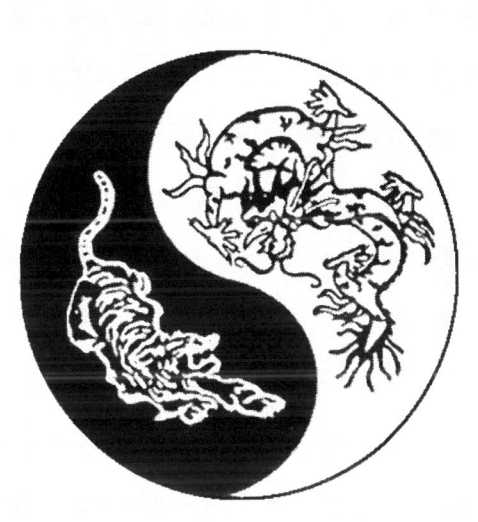

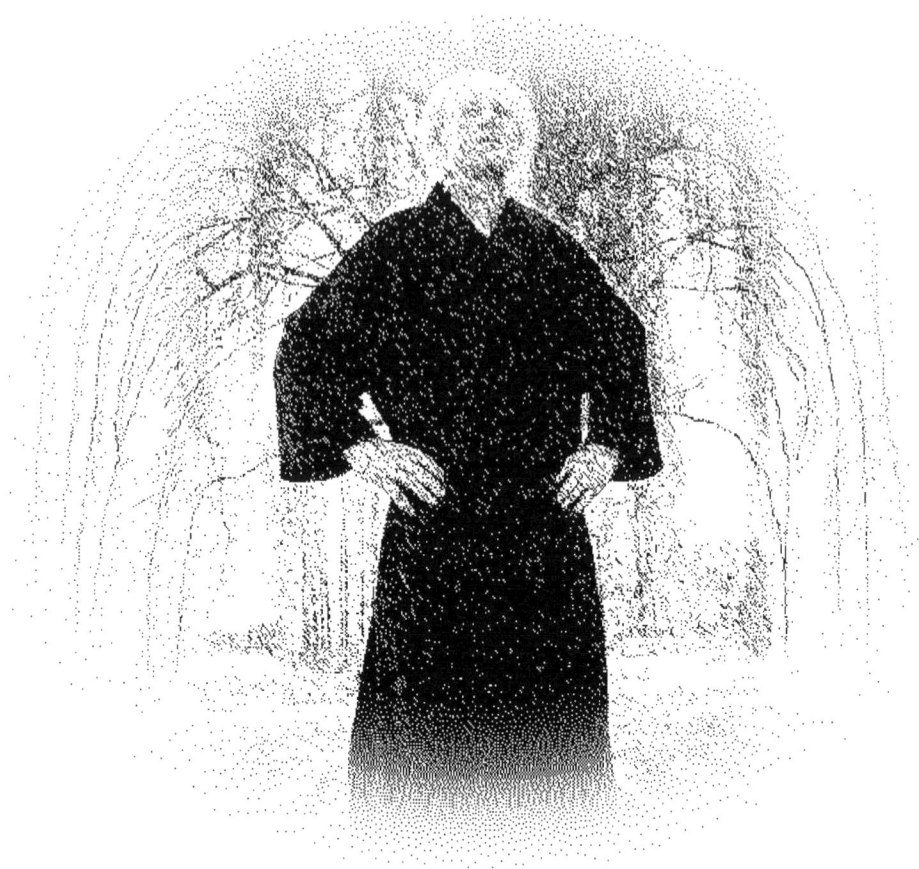

Others are revolted, I am unmoved.
Others are gripped by desires, I am unmoved.
Hearing the wisdom of sages, I am unmoved.
I move only in my own way.

These words were written by the Chinese poet Lu Yu in the 12th century. They were attributed to Bodhidarma. These words indicate one who has released all attachments and has become an Immortal Bodhisattva. Orientated from a perspective of Spirit, he now moves as Spirit.

Orientation — SHAOLIN TRADITION

At the foundation of all great religions and theosophies is the same Ultimate Truth that each religion and each seeker of Truth attempts to understand, live by and experience. Aspects of this Ultimate Truth recognized by all the great religions and seekers in one form or another are: Spirit Consciousness, Immortality, Omnipotence, Omniscience, Omnipresence, Love, Light, Compassion, Wisdom, Joy, Peace, Unity. These are all aspects of the Great Spirit, God, or what ever name it is given: Jehovah, Allah, Brahma, Ishvara, Tao, Amen-Ra, the list is almost endless. These are not different Gods. They are different words, used in different languages, for the same concept; the same God, the God of humanity and all of creation. The differences arise from misinterpretation of the teachings when they are disseminated. The experience of this Ultimate Truth is called by the different traditions: salvation, samadhi, satori, enlightenment, self realization, cosmic consciousness, Christ consciousness, etc..

All of the really great teachers of humanity taught virtually the same methods of obtaining this experience. They said that we cannot have this experience of Ultimate Truth without incorporating all the aspects of the Great Spirit into our own consciousness. This requires purification of our personality. The second requirement is that this experience can only be apprehended through our intuition. The vast majority of humans do not have intuitional ability strong enough to accomplish this. So the teachers gave us consciousness energization methods that would enable us to raise our intuitional ability to the levels required. Because our intuition is used, it is called mysticism. These time tested methods have been passed down to us by generations of highly advanced monks for literally thousands of years. They are compatible with the practices of all the great religions of the world.

Seekers within the Shaolin Tradition recognize the oneness of all people, of life, of creation, and attempt to realize the aspects of Truth for themselves. The tradition also involves itself with the dissemination of the teachings in the hope of one day achieving world peace and harmony. Throughout the history of this tradition it has acknowledged and used methods of achieving these goals from any effective source. It is recognized that Truth is at the core of all the great religions of the world. It was and is the norm for its seekers to participate in the activities of one or several other traditions. It has been said that a seeker in this tradition "may adhere to all, yet be bound by none". This occurred in the creation of the tradition.

The Shaolin Tradition began in the 6th century A.D., when an Indian kshatriya (member of the Hindu mediator caste) and Buddhist priest, came from India, to teach at the Shaolin Temple in China. This was the super sage Bodhidharma, his name in Sanskrit means "Wisdom Way". As a fully enlighten master, trained as a Kshatriya and a Buddhist Priest, he blended Hindu and Buddhist mysticism to create the Shaolin Tradition. This is why so many Sanskrit words and words with Sanskrit roots, are used within the Shaolin Teachings. At the temple he taught: personality purification (The Five Perfections), meditation, ayurvedic healing methods, martial methods and the consciousness energization methods of Vajramukti Yoga. This is the source of the teachings and methods used for the development of the foundation upon which the Shaolin Tradition evolved.

During the fifteen centuries that have followed, this tradition of methods of holistic human development has continued to evolve, with the ultimate goal of producing high levels of spiritual awareness for its practitioners and assisting in the eventual enlightenment of humanity.

Hindu Influence

Rishis are saints of prehistoric India who taught the yogic traditions, which included the Hindu yogic traditions for the development of spiritual awareness, ayurvedic health maintenance and medicinal techniques. It was the yogic teachers of India who traveled to China repeatedly through the centuries and brought the knowledge that the Shaolin Tradition is based on.

Pantanjali (900-800 B.C.) is the yogic saint that compiled the Yoga Sutras. It discussed yogic methods used to promote human development and spiritual growth. This classic outlined a scientific method of holistic development which had a profound influence on the development of both Buddhism and Taoism.

Mahavatar Babaji (November 30, 203 A.D. Considered an Immortal Bodhisattva) He is a raja Yoga Siddha. Babaji is known as the disseminator of the Kriya Yoga teachings (personality purification and consciousness energization methods) and Meditation. He assists humanity in its spiritual evolution.

Bodhidharma, (440 A.D. Considered an Immortal Bodhisattva) Founder of the Shaolin Tradition. Bodhidarma incorporated into the Shaolin Tradition his Hindu training as a Kshatriya. This influence included the teaching of meditation, consciousness energization methods, Vajra Mukti Yoga and much more (see Bodhidharma Background page 1 - 4) .

The Taoist influence

Lao-Tzu (1122-934 B.C.) is the Chinese sage who is given credit as the founder of Taoism. He wrote the original Taoist text The Tao Te Ching. Lao-Tzu was trained by the Indian siddha Boganathar.

Taoism is an indigenous philosophy of China. It may have been taught and practiced in China for 1500 years before Bodhidharma came to China. Historical researchers say that it can take less than 200 years for the practice of a philosophy or religion to become corrupted from the original teaching. By the time Buddhism was introduced to China, Taoism had been practiced for possibly over a 1000 years. By the time Buddhism was introduced, many devout Taoists had become frustrated with the Taoist priests for the excessive pomp and pageantry of ceremony performance and charging exorbitant fees for presiding over ceremonies such as holy festivals, marriages, and funerals. The mysticism of Buddhism and Taoism is very similar. In China and India, there is very little stigmatism involving the practice of more than one spiritual tradition at a time, as there is in Christianity. Many of the Taoists, not wanting to be associated with the Taoism any longer, became Buddhists. Through the centuries of operation of the Shaolin Temple, a large number of the monks and priests were both Taoist and Buddhist. This is why the Taoist influence at the Shaolin Temple, which is considered Buddhist, is so great.

Taoist knowledge and philosophy had a key role in the development of the Shaolin Tradition. Many of the nature concepts and imagery that are part of the Shaolin Tradition came from this Taoist influence. Examples are: The Tiger and Dragon, The Five Animals, The Five Elements, even the words chi and T'ai Chi have Taoist origins.

Buddhist influence

Siddhartha Gautama (563-483 B.C.) The Buddha, founder of Buddhism (also known as the Universal Religion). He taught the Yogic mysticism and ideals in what he called The Eight Fold Path and The Five Commands of Uprightness with an emphasis on non-violence.

The physical proximity and the relationship of the doctrine made this influence inevitable. The physical proximity of the Tibetian Buddhist center and one of the four main Shaolin Temples (this one in Yun-Nan Province of China, is on the border of Tibet) made them neighbors.

Bodhidharma, (440 A.D. Considered an Immortal Bodhisattva) Founder of the Shaolin Tradition, 28th Patriarch of Buddhism, 1st Patriarch of the Chan Buddhist Sect. In addition to this Buddhist influence, Bodhidarma incorporated into the Shaolin Tradition his Hindu training as a Kshatriya. This influence included the teaching of meditation, consciousness energization methods and much more (see Bodhidharma Background page 1 - 4).

Shaolin Influence

Shaolin Priest Yue, (about 1200 A.D.) According to legend, the Shaolin Master, Priest Yue, was the founder of the Yue Chia System. Priest Yue is also given credit for making the principles of the Thirteen Postures of T'ai Chi available to the Shaolin Priest Chang San Feng through the form Pai She Chuan (Form of the Ancient Wisdom of the White Snake).

Shaolin Master Priest Chang Sang Feng, (April 9, 1247 Considered an Immortal Bodhisattva) The Priest Chang San Feng is recognized as the originator of T'ai Chi. It was the Priest Chang San Feng that combined the Shaolin movements, mudra and Shaolin principles of the Snake and Crane to create T'ai Chi Chuan.

Shaolin Master Eizo Onishi, (1929 to present) Founder of Ken Do Gaku the Scientific Way. This Shaolin Master has made much of the esoteric knowledge of the Shaolin Tradition available to us.

Bodhidarma Background

      Saints and sages from India went to China repeatedly through the centuries teaching Buddhism and the Yogic Traditions. One of these saints was the super sage Bodhidharma. He was born in 440 A.D., his transition date is unknown. He is considered by many to be an Immortal Bodhisattva. His name in Sanskrit means "Wisdom Way". He is known as Ta-Mo in China and as Daruma in Japan. He was born a prince, son of the king Tamil Pallava of Kanchipuram. This made him a Kshatriya, born into the mediator caste of India. He took the vows and initiation into the Buddhist priesthood. His Buddhist teacher was Prajnatara, the 27th Indian Patriarch of Buddhism. Bodhidharma is considered the 28th Patriarch of Buddhism. Also, Bodhidarma is the 1st Patriarch of the Ch'an Buddhist Sect which became known as Zen in Japan.

      As a Kshatriya, Bodhidharma was trained in the classic arts of India: religion, esoterica, philosophy, literature, history, medicine, martial arts of India, Hindu mysticism and became a master of the esoteric methods of Vajramukti Yoga. Bodhidharma realized the abilities that the training of the Kshatriya so highly developed (Love, Peace, Compassion, Joy, morality, integrity, discipline, discernment, will, objectivity, concentration, intuition, etc.), were the very abilities that are prerequisite for spiritual realization.

      As a priest Bodhidharma was recognized as the 28th Patriarch of Buddhism because he taught meditation as a return to the original Buddhist Precepts. He was responsible for creating the Chan Buddhist Sect. Within Chan Buddhism, he blended Hindu and Buddhist mysticism and made meditation the primary tool for the development of spiritual awareness. This is why so many Sanskrit words and words with Sanskrit roots, are used within the Shaolin Teachings.

      Bodhidharma traveled to the Shaolin Temple in China in 520 A.D. and became recognized as the founder of the Shaolin Tradition. There he wrote the texts <u>Muscle/Tendon Changing</u> and <u>Marrow/Brain Washing</u>, which are the classics on the physical preparation for the development of spiritual awareness and consciousness energization. Four of his sermons have been preserved and handed down through the centuries: The Outline of Practice, The Bloodstream Sermon, The Wake-up Sermon, The Breakthrough Sermon.* At the temple he taught: personality purification (The Five Perfections), meditation, ayurvedic healing methods, martial methods and Vajramukti Yoga. Bodhidharma also taught the Vajramukti consciousness energization exercises which included Sanzan (Trican in Sanskrit), Crane breath, Cobra Breath and meditation. This is the source of the foundational methods upon which the Shaolin Tradition has evolved.

* These are available in English in a book called <u>The Zen Teaching of Bodhidaharma</u>
   ISBN 0-86547-399-4. It is required reading for all Shaolin Monastics.

Foundational Precepts

The teachings of Bodhidharma form the foundation of the Shaolin Tradition. Some of the foundational precepts of these teachings are:

that each of us are responsible for the development of our own spiritual awareness,
that at the source-core of our beings we are Spirit (the Supreme Consciousness),
that suffering is rooted in the ignorance of the awareness that we are Spirit,
that the experience of Spirit will end all stress and suffering,
that the amount of spiritual awareness one has, is directly proportional to the amount of energy that is available to ones consciousness,
that chi kung / pranayama, movement and meditation can be used to raise energy levels and bring a direct experience of Spirit,
that the teachings and methods presented within the this tradition are scientific, because if they are tested with sincerity, determination and discipline, they will work and prove to be true.

Aspects of Shaolin Tradition Introduced by Bodhidharma

Bodhidharma is the source of the Hindu and Buddhist influence within the Shaolin Tradition. Important aspects of Shaolin Tradition introduced by Bodhidharma are:

the use of meditation to develop spiritual awareness,
the use of the consciousness energization methods to enhance meditation ability,
the synergistic use of the three aspects of our being (physical, mental, spiritual) to enhance the holistic training and development of the individual,
the martial medium for use in the physical, mental and spiritual training,
the use of mudra to enhance the dissemination of spiritual knowledge and experience, and stimulate the motivation of the practitioners,
the use of forms as a medium to present and practice the use of mudra,
   Examples are San Zan Chuan, Sei San Chuan, San Sei Chuan, Bodhisattva Dao,
   Wu Hsing Chuan, Wu Shi Si, Pai She Chuan, Pai He Chuan
   (Also from the influence of Bodhidharma is the prolific use of mudra in the Shaolin T'ai Chi forms. They are: the 108, the Snake Form, the Form of the Five Elements, the Double Edged Sword Form, the Crane Form, and the Saber Form)
the use of *concepts of the worldly paradigm, contrasted with spiritual perception* to enhance the development spiritual awareness.

Orientation — Bodhidharma Background (continued)

There are seven hsing used for monk training at the Shaolin Temple in Westland Michigan. Three of those seven are the original three used by Bodhidharma to teach his first monks at the Shaolin Temple. They are San Zan Chuan, San Sei Chuan, and Sei San Chuan. These three hsing come from the Vajramukti Hindu sect of kundalini yogic mysticism. They are very ancient and could predate Bodhidharma by many centuries even millennia. The pranayamic methods that these hsing are based on are even older, perhaps dating into prehistory. The length of time that they have been practiced attests to their effectiveness.

These hsing have several purposes:

1) develop physical strength for the stamina required for meditation.
2) enhance mental abilities to comprehend concepts, techniques and methods used to develop spiritual awareness.
3) raise energy levels to develop the intuition, to enhance the results of meditation.
4) to develop concentration ability (dharana). Dharana is concentration with one pointed focused attention. This is required for efficient intuitional ability and meditation ability.
5) teach spiritual concepts through the mudra within the hsing, to speed up the process of the developing spiritual awareness.
6) build and sustain motivational levels so that the results of the training can be realized.
7) Samasthana training. Samasthana is self examination/personality purification used to expose the sthana to the self. The sthana is the personality; its belief system (including its limitations, delusions and illusions) and the resulting thought and behavior patterns.
8) develop the confidence and ability required to efficiently function as a mediator.

Orientation   Bodhidharma Background (continued)   1 - 7
Some Concepts with Which Bodidarma Was Familiar

The Six Paramitas (Six Virtues) as taught by Bodhidarma
This is originally a Hindu Metaphor.

The Six Paramitas of the sailboat that will carry one to the other shore.
This refers to crossing the sea of delusion (the worldly paradigm) to the other shore.
The other shore is a metaphor for Spiritual Realization.
All six must be practiced with perfect non-attachment from the perspective of performer and beneficiary.
The Five Perfections are the first five Paramitas.
Wisdom and Joy are the result of the practice of the Five Perfections.

1) Perfect Compassion and Charity refers to the emptiness within the interior of the boat
   without which a boat cannot float
2) Perfect Love and Morality refers to the keel.
   The keel is the spine of the boat. The spine is the source of its being.
3) Perfect Determination and Patience refers to the hull.
   The strength of the hull must be able to withstand the storms in the sea of delusion.
4) Perfect Discipline and Effort refers to the mast.
   The mast, in its upright position, stands at supreme attention placing
   Discipline and Effort at the forefront of consciousness.
5) Perfect Meditation and Spiritual Realization refers to the sail.
   The sail delivers the energy and insight from Spirit to the awareness of consciousness.
6) Wisdom and Joy refers to the tiller.
   The tiller gives appropriate direction and motivation to the consciousness.

The Four Skillful Actions of Bodhidarma
as described in his sermon, the "Entering the Buddha's Path ".
These are a variation of the Four Noble Truths of Buddhism.

1) Suffering Injustice
2) Adapting to Conditions
3) Desire Nothing (non-attachment)
4) Practicing the Dharma (the Dharma is the Five Perfections)

These are the **Four Noble Truths** of Buddhism:

1) All existence is marked by stress and suffering
2) Stress and suffering has a cause
3) The cause can be brought to an end
4) There is a way to end stress and suffering

1 - 8   Orientation   **Bodhidharma Background** (continued)
Some Concepts with which Bodhidarma was Familiar (continued)

The **Eightfold Noble Path** of Buddhism

1) Right Views
2) Right Purpose
3) Right Speech
4) Right Conduct
5) Right Livelihood
6) Right Spiritual Discipline
7) Right Awareness
8) Right Zen (meditation)

Heaven and Hell   **This is originally a Hindu Metaphor.**

Hell is considered an absence of spiritual realization (the Buddha Nature). Without spiritual realization one is subject to karma, stress and suffering. Hell is not a specific place. Heaven is the experience of spiritual realization: Immortality, Infinite Divine: Love, Light, Compassion, Truth, Wisdom, Joy, Peace and Bliss, etc.. This is an absence of all stress and suffering.
Life on Earth can be Heaven or hell depending on how much spiritual realization one has.

The Three Poisons are the **klesas**,   **This is originally a Hindu Metaphor.**

The Three Klesas are the psychologic demons that create all stress and suffering (all delusion) they are: self centeredness, fear, spiritual ignorance. All delusive thought and behavior manifest from the Three Klesas (hate, jealousy, greed, anger, avarice, attachment, etc.)

Zen

Zen is originally a Hindu concept. Zen is complete awareness of our Buddha Nature.
The Buddha Nature is the source-core of our being.
The source-core of our being is Supreme Consciousness, Spirit/God, the Buddha Nature.
Zen is the direct experience of the Supreme Reality; also synonymous with Spirit.
The experience of Zen results in complete awareness of Buddha Nature. The no-mindedness of the Buddha Nature is synonymous with Total Clarity and the Buddha Mind.
Bodhidarma also refereed to the process of obtaining the experience of Zen, as Zen.
Wu hsin is no-mindedness, the meditational state in which an experience of Zen can be obtained.
Bodhidarma also said that the Zen experience could occur spontaneously in a normal state of consciousness.

Orientation — Bodhidharma Background (continued)
Some Concepts with which Bodhidarma was Familiar (continued)

The Ten Precepts; include injunctions against:

Lay Buddhists
1) Murder and any physical assault on another
2) Theft
3) Adultery
4) Falsehood
5) Intoxication

Devout Buddhists   first 5 + these 3
6) Bodily adornment
    (ex. jewelry, tattoo, clothing that is too flattering)
7) Bodily comfort
    (ex. sleeping in a bed that is too soft)
8) Overeating
    (and eating after the noon meal)

Monks and Nuns   first 8 + these 2
9) Over indulgence in entertainment
10) Over indulgence in wealth

The Three Vows The Precepts are included and summarize the vows:

1) Injunction against evil and over indulgence in worldly behavior.
    Vow for the Lay Buddhists
2) Cultivate virtue
    Vow for Devout Buddhists includes Vow 1 and 2
3) Liberate all beings
    Vow for Monks and Nuns includes all 3 Vows

The Ten Good Deeds, is the avoidance of the ten evil deeds.
    Summarized by the maxim "Cause no suffering".

1) Murder and Maiming
2) Theft
3) Adultery
4) Falsehood
5) Slander
6) Profanity
7) Gossip
8) Avarice
9) Anger
10) Advocating false views

1 - 10   **Orientation   Bodhidharma Background** (continued)   **Bodhidharma Stories**

There are stories of Bodhidarma meditating for nine years in a cave staring at a rock wall. The nine years symbolize the length of time it takes to experience enlightenment if you are a sincere, determined, disciplined, initiated seeker. The wall symbolizes the worldly paradigm and the physical, astral, and causal veils that block our experience of Spirit. One's awareness must burn through this wall with the power of highly trained focused concentration and an indomitable will to experience Spirit. Bodhidarma was fully enlightened before he went to China. Meditation is a tool used to become enlightened. Once the goal is achieved, the tool is no longer required.

Another popular story is about Bodhidharma cutting off his eyelids so he could stay awake while meditating. He most probably used the Unmani Mudra while teaching meditation (using the Unmani Mudra, the eyelids are held half open). He did not really cut off his eyelids. The same story continues with Bodhidharma throwing his eyelids on the ground, where tea leaves sprouted, and were from then on used to make tea to help the monks stay awake while they were meditating. He is credited with introducing tea from India to China.

The story of Bodhidharma's departure from the Shaolin Temple is quite humorous. He had probably spent a little over ten years at the Temple training the monks and priests and setting up the foundation of the Shaolin Tradition. When he had accomplished his mission he prepared to go back to India. But during his stay at the Temple one of the leading monks had become very jealous of him, to the point of plotting Bodhidharma's murder. At this time Bodhidharma was approaching ninety, already almost three times the average life span for most of the people of that time. He had reached an age where a natural death looked emanate. The monk wanted the murder to look like the death was due to natural causes so he plotted to poison him. Since Bodhidharma was already an enlightened master, his intuition easily tipped him off to the plot. He realized that the intense guilt and shame the would be murderer would suffer, would probably move him to give up his worldly paradigm and dramatically assist the development of his spiritual awareness. He decided to let the monk think that he had accomplished his murderous task and allow the priests to inter his body in a tomb. When the funeral ceremonies were over Bodhidharma opened the tomb, intentionally left one of his sandals, then closed it behind him and left for India; not telling anyone. With his intuition, on the trail back to India at Northern Wei Pamair Heights, he manifested a meeting with a traveling government official by the name of Ambassador Song Yun. Bodhidharma knew that the Ambassador would mention to the monks at the Shaolin Temple that he had met Bodhidarma on the trail. He also knew that the official would tell the monks that it was peculiar that Bodhidharma was carrying only one sandal on his staff. Later the curious monks opened the tomb and found only one sandal, confirming to them that Bodhidharma had not died. After the guilty monk's lesson had achieved its goal, this news allowed him to become aware that he had not actually killed Bodhidharma. This relieved some of the guilt and shame, making his life livable again and eventually enabled him to give up the worldly paradigm and achieve satori. This story was probably preserved as evidence of Bodhidharma's status as an Immortal Bodhisattva. This empty tomb of Bodhidharma still exists near Loyang at the Tinglin Temple on Bear Ear Mountain.

Kshatriya; Ethics and Influence

Kshatriya is the Hindu warrior caste of India within which Bodhidarma was born. The mainstream use of the term warrior caste is really incorrect. It is really a caste of mediators. The primary duty of the Kshatriya was to keep the peace within their society. They would mediate conflicts between individuals and groups.

Without exception the Kshatriya were expected to adhere to the principle of Dharmavijaya, the law of righteous behavior and the righting of wrongs or injustices encountered, irrespective of who committed them. These are some of the rules that guided the behavior of the Kshatriya that are mentioned in the Bhagavad Gita. These rules are still used for guidance of Shaolin trained monks.

- Those who attack by the use of words should only be fought with words.
- If violence is required it must be used only to the point necessary to secure the safety of all those involved.
- One should only strike when necessary in response to an attack or after giving options, warning and due notice.
- One fighting another person should not be attacked.
- A Kshatriya should not strike one who is tired, weeping, unwilling to fight, who is ill, or who cries surrender.
- A Kshatriya should defend even an enemy who has surrendered with folded hands.
- In war, civilians are to be allowed to continue their life unhindered.
- Temples and places of worship are not to be touched.
- A Kshatriya should never strike a priest, for by doing so he attacks his own source.

Trained in religion, esoterica, philosophy, literature, history, ayurvedic medicine and martial arts, the Kshatriya served as healers, social workers and mediators. They served the same function and were part of the same social structure as the Judges of the Old Testament (here is a tie to the Judeao-Christian Tradition). Trained in the classic arts of the Kshatriya, Bodhidarma became a master of the esoteric methods of Vajramukti. Vajramukti is a mystical yogic sect of spiritual development used by many Kshatriya. Vajramukti training included: physical training used for preparation for the spiritual training, the Personality Purification Methods, meditation, the Consciousness Energization Methods used to develop the intuition and enhance the results of meditation, and the psycho-physical exercises (chi-kung/ pranayama, forms training) used to enhance the spiritual training.

Bodhidharma used the Kshatriya training and their goals as a template for the design of the monk training at the Shaolin Temple. The Shaolin ideals of social service came from the Hindu Kshatriya. He expected the Shaolin trained monks to act as spiritual mediators within the Chinese culture. Through Love and Compassion, the Shaolin Monks were trained to disseminate the spiritual teachings of mysticism to humanity and assist humanity in maintaining the Peace. The monk's heightened intuitional abilities were used not only to enhance their meditation and thereby develop their spiritual awareness, but also to enhance their ability to serve humanity as healers, social therapists and counselors, just as the Kshatriya were expected to do. This is the source of the goals and methods used for the spiritual training at the Shaolin Temple; the foundation upon which the Shaolin Tradition has evolved.

1 - 12   Orientation   Comments of Master Sensei Eizo Onishi
Areas of Self Development, Aspects of Spirit,
Aspects of Physical Fitness, Aspects of Health

Areas of Self Development:

1) spiritual - character, morality, awareness of Spirit (see below)

2) physical - technique, health

3) mental - ability to concentrate, self discipline, knowledge, recall ability, objectivity in thought, intuitional ability, etc.

Aspects of Spirit: of which we develop an awareness of within ourselves

1) Love 2) Truth 3) Peace 4) Unity 5) Omnipresent

6) Light 7) Wisdom 8) Bliss 9) Immortality 10) Omnipotent

11) Life 12) Joy 13) The Word 14) Freedom 15) Omniscient

16) Infinite 17) Creator 18) Ultimate All

"Ye are Gods". - Jesus   John 10: 34

Aspects of Physical Fitness:
developed to enhance our mental faculties and our physical ability to interact with the world.

1) speed, quickness 4) timing 6) precision

2) coordination 5) balance 7) flexibility

3) agility 6) stamina 9) strength

Aspects of Health:

1) hygiene
2) sleep - appropriate duration and regularity of time
3) exercise
4) nutrition - balanced meals - proper amount - supplements
5) herbology - for health, vitality and medication
6) chi kung - massage - acupressure - physical and mental energization
7) meditation

Leaders   Master Sensei Eizo Onishi

History has shown the great influence that leaders have on their students. The best leaders are those who expend the most effort on their students, and who are capable themselves of changing as a result of their efforts.

Slavish imitation is the method of primitive people. Rather than insist on mere imitation, good leaders are those who give Light to their students, helping them with their own creative thinking. The instances in which they insist that something is absolutely correct are very few. Leaders must never forget that the learning and study process must be continuous until the goal is achieved.

Comments on Discipline

The purification of thought patterns and behavior that paralyze growth is possible if one follows a path of self discipline. Techniques are not enough to produce expansion of awareness.

Only direct experience is legitimate knowledge. Control of the mind cannot be accomplished without self discipline, and without control of the mind, direct experience is not possible.

It is imperative that a life of self discipline be adhered to. There needs to be a connection between the life within and the life without. Discipline is the source of that connection.

Self discipline will enable self discovery and self discovery will enable direct experience. Direct experience will expand your awareness. Expansion of awareness is the purpose of life.

Shiva
The Source of Change
King of the Yogis
The Disseminator of Yogic Knowledge

"For everyone shall be salted with fire, and every sacrifice shall be salted with salt.
Salt is good: but if the salt have lost his saltiness, where with will ye season it?
Have salt in yourselves, and have peace one with another."
　　　　　　　　　　　　　　　　　　　　　　　- Jesus

The Fish Asking About Water
        As told by Yogacharya, Sri John Oliver Black

    Some fish were having a discussion one day about what water was. As the fish discussed water, they noted that in their environment, water was perfectly clear and it seemed to have no weight. Any odors or color in the water seemed to come from something in the water and not the water its self. As the fish moved in the water, there did not seem to be anything there to touch. The discussion seemed very metaphysical to them because they could not seem to see, feel, smell or touch it with any certainty. They eventually came to the conclusion that they needed help to even ascertain the reality of water.

    One of the fish mentioned that he knew of a very wise fish that might be able to shed some light on the subject. So the fish decided to make the trip to find the wise fish and if they found him they would ask him if he knew anything about water. The fish had to travel a great distance and overcome many obstacles. But, due to their sincerity, determination and discipline, they eventually found the wise fish and obtained an audience with him.

    The fish were able to describe their dilemma about water to the wise fish. The wise fish responded saying that all fish: breath, eat, play, and sleep in it, obtain energy from it and experience their life in water. He told them that they were even made of the water they were in. He explained that their five senses were not developed enough to apprehend and experience water so that they could have direct knowledge of it. The wise fish continued saying that the only way they could apprehend and experience water, was to develop their sixth sense, intuition. Then to use their intuition to look deeply into their own self for the direct experience of water as the ocean, that they themselves are.

    Just as humans are Immortal Beings of Spirit, existing in the Ocean of Spirit.

Comparison of Moral Codes and Discipline

The Buddhist; Eight Fold Path
Consists of aligning the self with God in eight areas of physical and mental activity.
1) Correct views
2) Correct purpose
3) Correct speech
4) Correct conduct
5) Correct vocation
6) Correct effort
7) Correct awareness (meditation)
8) Correct concentration
    (God Communion)

The Five Buddhist Commands of Uprightness
1) Do not kill
2) Do not steal
3) Do not lie
4) Do not commit adultery
5) Do not become intoxicated

6 Paramitas of Hinduism and Buddhism:
1) Perfect Compassion develops Perfect Charity
2) Perfect Love develops Perfect Morality
3) Perfect Determination develops Perfect Patience
4) Perfect Discipline develops Perfect Effort
5) Perfect Concentration/Meditation
   Once the first four perfections are incorporated into the personality then Perfect meditation will result in Illumination
6) Illumination will result in Perfect Wisdom and Perfect Joy

The Hindu; The Eight Limbs of Raja Yoga
1) Yama   self restraint
2) Niyama   self discipline
3) Asana   posture
4) Pranayama   breath control
5) Pratyahara   sense control
6) Dharana   concentration
7) Dhyana   meditation
8) Samadhi   God communion

Purification of the Personality

Energization of Consciousness

Taoist Yoga; Alchemy of Eight Stages to Salvation
1) Conservation of Essence
2) Restoration of Essence
3) Transmutation of Essence
4) Nourishing the Chi (prana)
5) Transmutation of Chi
6) Nourishing the Shen (soul)
7) Transmuting Shen (meditation)
8) Transmuting Void (God communion)

Yama; 5 restraints
1) non-violence
2) truthfulness
3) non-stealing
4) sensual control
5) non-possessiveness

Niyama; 5 observances
1) purity
2) commitment
3) spiritual exercise
4) self study
5) contentment

Taoist Stage 1
Conservation of Essence requires the Hindu 5 restraints

Taoist Stage 2
Restoration of Essence requires the Hindu 5 observances

1 - 16   Orientation   **The Shaolin Tradition Genealogy from Bodhidharma**

Kong Su Kung - Chinese Shaolin Master
 Chinese Ambassador to Okinawa
 Taught Shaolin Tradition
    to Okinawan's

↓

Tode Sakugawa: 1733-1815 (Okinawan)
 Taught Kushanku Kata;
 Taught to him by Kong Su Kung
    Also studied in Fukien

↓

Sobi (Sokon) Matsumura "Bushi"
 Okinawan Master 1796-1893;
    Also studied in Fukien

↓

From here on, the arts of this line are called
 Shuri-te and **Shorin-ryu**

↓

Itosu Ankoh (Yasutsune) 1828-1915
 Okinawan Shaolin Master,
 created the five Pinan Kata.

↓

Kanken Toyama 1888-1967
 Okinawan, Shaolin Master,
 President of the first
    All Japan Karate-Do Federation

Bai Yi Feng: circa 1300 A.D. Shaolin Master
 Founder of Wuzuquan (Five Ancestor's Fist Way)
 Taught Southern Shaolin, including:
    Bodhidarma's teaching's

↓

Chatan Yao "Yara" circa 1700 A.D. (Okinawan)
 Studied in Fukien Province of China.
 Taught Fukien arts in Okinawa.

↓

Woo Lu Chin, Chinese, Shaolin Master
    (Okinawan name; Ryo Ryu)
 Taught Fukien arts including Wuzuquan

↓

From here on, the arts of this line are called
 Naha-Te and **Shorei-Ryu**

↓

Kanryo Higashionna 1849-1915
 Okinawan Shaolin Master
 Studied in Fukien, Fukien arts only

↓

Juhatsu Kyoda 1888-1966
 Okinawan, Shaolin Master
 Founded Toon-Ryu, Chief instructor
    of the Dai Nippon Butoku Kai

↓   ↓

Eizo Onishi; 1929
    Japanese Shaolin Master
Shue Cheng Zhi →   Shiohan Dai of Toyama
 Chinese, Shaolin Master   Founder of Koeikan Ken Do Gaku
 Taught: Vajra Mukti Yoga, Chuan Fa,
 Shaolin T'ai Chi, Yue Chia Kung fu

                    Yogacharya Sri John Oliver Black,
                    1893 - 1989 Enlightened Yoga Master
Richard Franks and Michael Brokas   Taught Raja Yoga and SRF Kriya Yoga
 T'ai Chi Chuan and T'ai Chi Chi-Kung   Direct disciple of Paramahansa Yogananda
                       and Babaji's line of Kriya Yoga Gurus

↓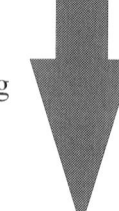

Thomas F. Smith, 1950: Founder of the Shaolin Temple of Michigan

1 - 17
Orientation
Historical Map

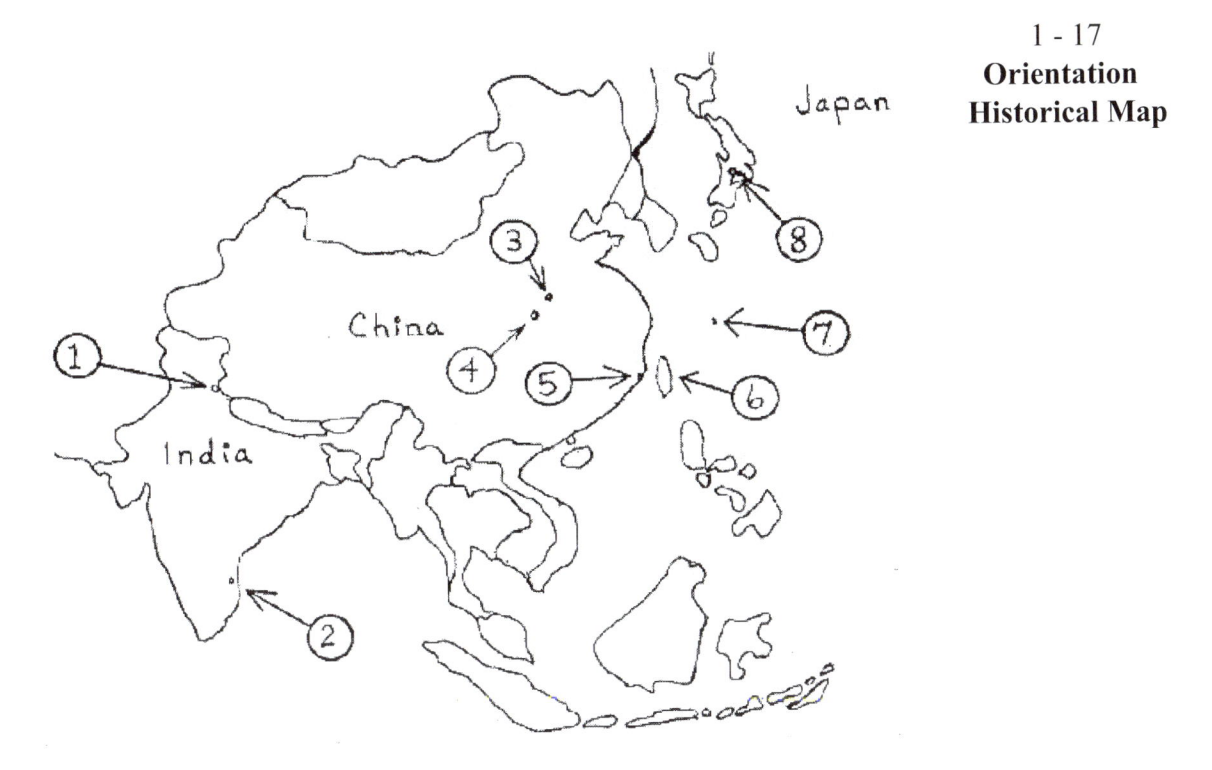

1) Cave of Babaji - near Badrinath, northern India. Babaji is the spiritual leader of the Kriya Yoga Tradition and a powerful force in the spiritual evolution of humanity.
2) Birthplace of Bodhidarma - Kancipura, southern India
3) The Honan Shaolin Temple - in the western Songshan mountains, Denfeng County, Honan Province. This is the first Shaolin Temple, where Bodhidarma originated the Shaolin Tradition. During the centuries that followed hundreds of minor Shaolin Temples were established in China. Eventually four main temples came into operation: 1) this one in Honan 2) the Wu Tang Temple 3) the Fukien Temple 4) the Yun-nan Temple (also known as the Hunan Temple), at the south China border near Tibet.
4) Wu Tang Mountain, Shaolin Temple - This is the site of the hermitage where the Shaolin Priest, Chang San Feng developed and taught the Shaolin Wu Tang Methods and T'ai Chi. This became one of the four main temples of the Shaolin Tradition on the mainland in China.
5) Southeastern Shaolin Temple of Fukien - in Putian, Fujian Province. This temple was built just a few generations after Bodhidarma left Honan. This temple lasted many centuries providing spiritual training in Bodhidarma's methods. It had great influence on the Okinawan arts.
6) Taiwan - Present center of the Shaolin Tradition. The communists on the Chinese mainland have been trying to eliminate all the ancient spiritual belief systems and organizations in China. They have tortured and murdered those that they could catch who would not give up their spiritual practices. Most of the Shaolin have moved to Taiwan.
7) Okinawa - Historically the island of Okinawa has been a stronghold for several groups that have retained and past on the Shaolin Tradition; including the spiritual training methods of Bodhidarma. These small groups have made a large contribution to the world martial arts culture. Some of these groups may still exist on Okinawa.
8) Yamato Dojo of Eizo Onishi - in Yamato, Japan, not far from Mount Fuji. This is the temple where the Shaolin Master, Eizo Onishi, taught the Shaolin Tradition.

Orientation — The Original Five Animal Methods of the Shaolin Tradition

The animal imagery is a direct result of the Taoist influence within the Shaolin Tradition. The mainstream understanding of these five animal categories is that they are different fighting styles, but actually they were different areas of knowledge. Some fighting techniques and strategies eventually became attributed to each of the animals but they were used to identify areas of study and training. All of these techniques and strategies were considered part of the original Shaolin style. They did become styles or systems of fighting when the knowledge and methods were made available to people outside of the Temple, people who did not have full understanding of the Shaolin Tradition. The areas of study and training and some of these techniques and strategies have been noted here.

Tiger

Since the power and ability of the Tiger seems supernatural, it is considered of the Realm of Spirit and its super power, metaphysical. It is fierce, courageous and powerful. The Tiger will maneuver to attack the most vulnerable position, usually the back or side. It attacks with overwhelming speed and power. These methods are used to train internal strength, to develop a strong immune system, spiritual awareness and the ability to use internal energy in the delivery of martial technique. The Tiger Claw (finger tips) is sometimes used for striking precision targets. It is also used to grab, to take control of attackers (neutralize attacks, expose targets, deliver throws).

The Tiger represents the Cosmic Creative Force of Yin and therefore Life. It represents Life in all its manifestations, both pleasant and unpleasant. It is the catalyst of positive change and evolution. As the Feminine Cosmic Creative Being of Creation, the Tiger can be invoked for spiritual assistance.

The Tiger is Yin to the Dragon.

Dragon

The Dragon does not have to stalk or plan its attack in any way. It relies on super power to instantly overwhelm its attacker as it moves with majesty and grace. The Dragon can appear out of nowhere, and it can disappear. It can bilocate and be everywhere at once.

The Dragon is the Cosmic Creative Force of Yang. It is considered to be a supreme divine spiritual creature, possessing the attributes of Spirit (omnipotence, omniscience, omnipresence, Love, Compassion, Light, Joy, Wisdom, Peace). It is the model for spiritual development. As the Masculine Cosmic Creative Being of Creation, the Dragon can be invoked for spiritual assistance.

The Tiger and Dragon are considered the creative aspect of the Great Spirit. They correlate to the Heavenly Father (Dragon), the masculine aspect of the Creator and the Divine Mother (Tiger) the feminine aspect of the Creator. It is the interaction of the Tiger and Dragon that is responsible for the manifestation of Creation and through this process, the cosmic sound of Om is generated.

The Dragon is Yang to the Tiger.

Orientation
Influence of the Original Five Animal Methods of the Shaolin Tradition (continued)

Snake

The Snake moves with speed and power by coordinating the use of as many muscle groups as possible as it performs each movement. It unwinds its body in a chain reaction as it develops its great speed and power. It is an expression of perfect balance since it stays so close to the ground. It goes in low even when it attacks. It knows how to wait for the most opportune moment and is good at the ambush. When it takes its attacker down it can wrap it up and crush its bones.

The Snake is considered the Earthly Dragon having the attributes of the Dragon but in the realm of the Earth. The Snake methods are used to develop the ability to use chi kung to develop spiritual awareness. The Cobra Snake symbolizes and even looks like the brain, medulla, and spinal cord. This is the cerebral spinal path used to energize the upper tan tien (the spiritual eye) and turn on the intuition. Intuition is humanity's the sixth sense, the only sense that will provide us with an experience of spirit. The technique used to energize the upper tan tien is called the Cobra Breath. Tamo's "Bone and Marrow Changing Methods" describe how chi kung can be used to develop spiritual awareness and are the foundation of The Shaolin Snake Methods.

The Snake is Yin to the Crane.

Crane

The Crane fights with speed, grace and agility. It is very light on its feet, changing direction rapidly and gyrating its body with perfect coordination. It develops power from speed and is able to deliver lighting fast, focused strikes. The Crane can fly in as it attacks and can be aggressive. It is likely to attack higher targets. The Crane will fight in close with its wings and long legs as the Shaolin Crane Methods will use fist, elbow, knee and foot techniques and in combinations.

The Crane is the symbol of Wisdom and the Crane Methods uses Chi Kung to develop physical and mental health. Tamo's "Muscle and Tendon Changing Methods" describe how chi kung can be used to do this and prepare the body for spiritual training. These methods are the foundation of The Shaolin Crane Methods.

The Crane is Yang to the Snake.

Orientation

Influence of the Original Five Animal Methods of the Shaolin Tradition (continued)

Panther

This is the Tiger of the Earth realm. Powerful, fast and agile, the Panther is the master of the stalk and economy of motion. Every movement, even its slightest movement, has purpose. It plans its approach in detail. It takes into consideration everything in the situation and environment. And can use its intellect and intuition to be novel and creative in completing its tasks.

The Panther is the model of self discipline and objectivity (the ability to perceive truth and use knowledge to come to appropriate conclusions). It has an acute awareness of its situation and circumstance; and is able to make the most of it. It uses no more than what is required. The panther assumes responsibility for its Life, thoughts and behavior; and takes control of its destiny. It seeks to achieve harmony with what it does and its environment; and achieves balance of the Yin and Yang.

Because it is of the realm of Earth it is born without cosmic knowledge. But at the core of its being it knows there is more to reality than what it can see, touch and smell. So it compensates by purifying its self and developing its intuition; and realizes and experiences itself, and its environment, as Spirit.

It can do this because it revels in its Life and chooses to allow Love, Wisdom and Joy to permeate its being.

The Panther is the template for holistic human development.

Difference Between a Warrior and a Soldier

Soldiers and many officers of the law, politicians and lawyers, do what they call their duty, because a powerful entity (usually the society they were born in, or a special interest group) gives them money and tells them what they are doing is morally right. They accept the money and usually do what they are told without really looking into the motives of this entity. Their moral orientation, which is usually influenced by family, culture and the laws of the land, determines what is morally right and wrong for them. They end up doing what they are told "doing their duty", blindly following orders; and often becoming a minion of greed obsessed, corrupt sociopaths.

In contrast to the soldier, the warrior is one who does what he or she does with full and detailed, self considered knowledge of what they do and why. They do not do what they are told to do, just because someone with "perceived" authority has told them something is so. They pledge their allegiance, consciously, to **self-decided** reasons for their thoughts and behavior; not social influences. They take full responsibility for all their thoughts and behaviors. For an immature personality with an undeveloped moral orientation, this also could be for a greed obsessed, corrupt sociopath. But for a Spirit Warrior, the self is seen as part of humanity, creation and Spirit. The thoughts and behaviors of a Spirit Warrior are aligned with and motivated by, what is good for All.

The 1st and 2nd Task; The Spirit Warrior becomes a Bodhisattva

As part of the All, the Spirit Warrior recognizes his influence on others in his immediate vicinity and on humanity at large. With this recognition, the Spirit Warrior recognizes that his or her primary task, even responsibility, is making that influence the best it can be. This orientation is motivated by an intuitionally perceived understanding of the self as Spirit. And as Spirit, is functioning with the Love and Compassion of Spirit. To make this influence the best it can be, the Spirit Warrior realizes that he or she must incorporate into his personality all the aspects of Spirit (Love, Light, Compassion, Truth, Wisdom, Joy, Peace, Bliss, etc.). This includes a highly developed intellect, and stable, balanced, controlled emotions. For Shaolin, this is achieved through the practice of meditation, the application of the Personality Purification Process and the Consciousness Energization Exercises of the Shaolin Tradition. Inner Peace and Joy (the elimination of personal suffering and fear) is the first step in developing ones positive influence. Efficient assistance to others can not be accomplished until substantial progress is made in this first step. The second task is to assist in the elimination of the suffering of others until all suffering is ended. This involves assisting all others in the complete development of their spiritual awareness. With acceptance of this second task, the Spirit Warrior becomes a Bodhisattva. A Bodhisattva has made this second task the primary goal of his or her existence.

Orientation — **The Spirit Warrior** (continued)

Responsibility for the Self

The Spirit Warrior must throughly acknowledge that we are totally responsible for all of our thoughts and behaviors: and all of our situations and circumstances. Once we are about 13 years old we have matured enough to be able to think in abstract terms and use symbolism in thought processes. The potential to understand cause and effect becomes dramatically enhanced. Even the rules and mechanics of karma become available to us if we are inquisitive and motivated. With this ability we can make more sense of our environment and interact more efficiently with it. Those that do not allow childhood conditioning and irrational emotion to control their thoughts, conclusions and behaviors, can train themselves to be objective and perceive Truth. We have, then, the potential to re-evaluate our previous conditionings and conclusions for appropriateness and make the changes that are required. This is Self-examination and Personality Purification in action. Freewill enables us to make choices. The choices that we make in our thoughts and behavior determine our situations and circumstances. When we use the required discipline to make the appropriate choices, we can direct the manifestation of what happens in our lives. Poor choices will produce stressful results. Appropriate choices will produce beneficial results. With this knowledge, we have the potential to take control of our lives. The Spirit Warrior knows that we are responsible for what happens to us and is capable of directing his or her own destiny.

Our time in the earth plane is really quite short. When our immortality is experienced, eighty years or so is a flash in the expanse of eternity. It is important to make the most of the time that we have here and to extend this time as long as possible. The physical body we have been given is like a tool we can use to interact with the environment of Earth. In order to be most efficient with the time we have, this tool must be taken care of the best that we can. Even the performance of our mental and intuitional abilities are directly influenced by the health and vitality levels of our physical body. Our bodies are sacred. They actually house an incarnation of Spirit. And our physical body is sometimes called a Temple of God. While we are here on Earth, the Spirit Warrior recognizes the value the body has to the mission we have embraced. The health and energy the body has available to it, has a direct impact on what can be accomplished during our time here. The best possible health regimens must be strictly adhered to, which include physical and mental energization exercises.

These exercises are performed not only for the physical body, but also to enhance the function of the mind. The human brain uses more energy than any other organ in the physical body. The mind cannot operate efficiently without high levels of vitality and energy. The Spirit Warrior trains the mind for sustained mental focus to enhance the efficiency of everything that is attempted. The daily regimen of consciousness energization exercises are required to obtain the energy levels necessary for the accomplishment of the task we have set for ourselves.

The weapons of the Spirit Warrior are the aspects of Spirit. The tools are the techniques of Personality Purification, Consciousness Energization, the 5 Perfections and *meditation*.

"What you call a temple we call a sangharama, a place of purity. But whoever denies entry to the three poisons (the klesic demons) and keeps the gates of his senses pure, his body and mind still, inside and outside clean, builds a temple."   - Bodhidarma

Orientation   The Spirit Warrior (continued)

Self Examination / Personality Purification   The Battlefield of the Spirit Warrior

The development of spiritual perception requires the purification of the personality. The depths of Truth and Reality can not be apprehended without the removal of all negativity and incorporating the aspects of Spirit (Love, Compassion, Truth, Wisdom, Joy, etc.) into the personality. This is Personality Purification. The practice of meditation will produce personality purification and is required, but this active procedure of Personality Purification will dramatically enhance the process. The Process of Personality Purification is the application of choice. It is an exercise of freewill. All thoughts and behavior are choices. If we choose to entertain negativity in any form (worldly perspective) it will attract more stress and suffering. If we choose to operate from an orientation of Spirit (perspective of Spirit) we will attract positive circumstances and Joy. This is the Cosmic Law of Karma. In the Process of Personality Purification, one is expected to monitor one's self for negative thoughts and behavior, attachments, immorality, rationalizations, denials, delusions, illusions, transferences, etc. and eliminate them. One must become completely non-violent, truthful, non-stealing, non-possessive, and not do anything that will overly reduce energy levels. Spiritual ignorance, narcissism, and fear must be completely eliminated.

When your own limitations are exposed to yourself, identified and analyzed for appropriateness, then, through:
    1) an act of will,
    2) a solemn commitment to the elimination of inappropriate thought, behavior and belief,
    3) and continued monitoring of one's thought and behavior for inappropriateness,
one can make the changes required to eliminate those limitations.

A choice and decision is made to end the repetition of the identified inappropriate thought and or behavior. All thoughts, biases, behaviors and beliefs must be evaluated for appropriateness and self-directed change must occur when called for. Predominate thoughts, beliefs and biases must be identified and paid special attention. All current beliefs are to be examined for validity and re-examined again as more information is obtained. This process is repeated until perfection is attained. Eventually, all thoughts and behavior will manifest from pure Spiritual Perception.

Summary and Suggestions

1) This method requires that all thoughts, biases, behaviors and beliefs (particularly beliefs that influence behavior) be examined for appropriateness and validity.
The criteria used should be based on Spiritual Perception versus worldly perception. Inappropriate behavior, belief, bias and thought are often accompanied by anxiety, depression, fear, guilt, anger, pride, etc. which can present a clue to inappropriateness.
2) All thoughts, beliefs, and behaviors must be evaluated for appropriateness and self directed change must occur if called for. A choice and decision is made to end the repetition of the identified inappropriate thought, behavior, and or change the invalid belief.
3) All current beliefs are to be examined for validity and re-examined again as more information is obtained. Again, self-directed change must occur when required.
4) This process is repeated until perfection is attained.

The Worldly Paradigm; Spiritual Ignorance

The goal (complete spiritual realization) must be pursued as if the Spirit Warrior is going into battle. For the Spirit Warrior, the battle is found within his or her own consciousness. It is there, where the demons of spiritual ignorance reside. The goal is obtained with the defeat of the klesic demons: self centeredness, fear, ignorance. It is spiritual ignorance that pollutes the consciousness, blocking our view of reality and Truth; and the development of our spiritual awareness. It is spiritual ignorance that creates the klesic demons and all the personality issues that come with them. *Spiritual ignorance is the result of the false beliefs and conclusions made in response to our experiences gained while living in the world.*

The tools we use to apprehend experience, are our five senses and intellect. These senses will give us information about what we can see, hear, touch, smell and taste in our environment. Using only our five senses, we are born, live and die accumulating information only about life on Earth. When the people around us die, we do not usually hear anything from them again. It looks as if their existence has ended. This is usually all the information that we have on which to base our understanding of reality. We might be told something different from what we experience, but it is hard to argue with the evidence. Even if we profess something different, our subconscious belief system is what we operate with. Unless we are blessed with some intuition, it appears that this is all that exists. However, there is so much more to reality that it cannot even be imagined. The evidence available to us from our five senses does not permit us to come close to apprehending accurate beliefs and conclusions about reality.

This ignorance produces the worldly paradigm of self centeredness, self obsession and fear. The worldly paradigm is the orientation to life where one believes and operates under the incorrect assumption that life in the world is separate from life in Spirit. This is the result of the subconscious or even conscious belief that our life on earth is all that we will have and that when we make our earthly transition our consciousness will end. It is the spiritual ignorance that is developed over the duration of our life that makes us believe that we are mere mortals. With this belief we think of ourselves as autonomous, separate from all others and total annihilation imminent. From this orientation of understanding, the situations and circumstances of what we believe is our short life, completely depend on our own efforts. There does not seem to be consequences for inappropriateness unless we are caught. Feelings of desperateness can lead us to ignore the law and the rules. There can be an overwhelming tendency to interact selfishly with others to obtain better circumstances and security. Our behaviors often become narcissistic and self centered, using the efforts of others without due compensation, blatantly causing suffering for others and unconsciously causing suffering for the self. These beliefs (the worldly paradigm, spiritual ignorance) will generate all negativity: insecurity, poor self-esteem, a low self concept, feelings of ineffectiveness and inability, self centeredness, self obsession, greed, jealousy, envy, anxiety, anger, fear, personal and global suffering.

Through Compassion and Love, the Spirit Warrior makes the end of global stress and suffering the mission of his or her life. A Spirit Warrior must become the Five Perfections and perfectly develop self purification and consciousness energization to defeat the klesic demons and achieve success. With the development of the Five Perfections (which includes daily meditation) the personality of the Spirit Warrior evolves into a Bodhisatva.

Orientation — The Spirit Warrior (continued)

Detachment

The Spirit Warrior must understand and practice detachment.

To understand detachment, attachment must be fully understood. Attachment is an attempt to gain happiness and security. Attachment is an emotional desire to possess and retain things that produce and maintain security and comfort. These things can be material items, thoughts and professed beliefs.

Change is an integral aspect of creation. Everything in creation is in constant change. Nothing in creation remains the same. The Creator intentionally designed it to operate in this way. This design has fundamental and foundational purpose. Change makes stress and suffering possible. The Creator's Plan uses stress and suffering to cultivate Compassion and Love in humanity. The search for the answer to the problem of stress and suffering leads to Love and Compassion, which results in Spiritual Perception. The purpose could not be achieved without change. Change creates the environment to entertain and teach. Stress and suffering are required to motivate the discovery of Spiritual Perception.

To take advantage of the Great Spirit's plan we have opted to experience creation. We are immortal spiritual beings whose immortality will not change. From the worldly paradigm, we are not very much aware of this. The worldly paradigm produces the belief in our mortality. The belief of our mortality creates insecurity. Insecurity will produce worldly thoughts and behavior, which in turn produces stress, fear and suffering. When our circumstances are comfortable we strive to maintain that comfort especially after we have experienced discomfort. We very often become obsessed with obtaining and maintaining security and comfort to the point of entertaining inappropriate thoughts and behaviors, which in turn produces more stress and suffering. This in turn produces attachment to things we feel will maintain our security and comfort, which very often becomes even more obsessive. Then the attachments produce stress and suffering from the fear of losing the attachment and from the effort involved in maintaining the possession of the attachment. When obsession develops, gluttony sets in, producing more stress and suffering. When change causes an attachment to fail to produce security and or comfort, the attempt to adapt to its loss results in another attachment. The process becomes a vicious cycle. All this is based on the delusion that our comfort and security can be maintained within creation by things, thoughts and professed beliefs. It is delusion because nothing within creation can stay the same for very long. Everything changes. The only thing that does not change is Spirit. Through Spiritual Perception we come to realize that at the core of our beings we are Spirit (Changeless, Infinite Love, Light, Truth, Wisdom, Joy, Peace and Bliss) and that this is the only source of complete and permanent security and comfort.

The Spirit Warrior acknowledges change and the results of change as an aspect of creation. Then makes a choice and decision to not develop attachments to anything within creation.

Bodhidharma said that "All appearances are illusion, do not hold on to appearances. If you seek direct understanding of Truth, do not hold on to any appearance whatsoever, and you will succeed." from the Bloodstream Sermon

Orientation — The Spirit Warrior (continued) — Truth, Will

Truth, Will - In order to obtain and provide positive influence on personal and global problems, the aspects of Spirit must be incorporated into the personality. Aspects such as Love and Compassion maybe obvious but the aspects of Truth, Will, Optimism, Gratitude, and Forgiveness may need addressing.

Truth - The development of spiritual awareness is proportionate to the level of the aspects of Spirit, that are incorporated into the personality. Since Truth is an aspect of Spirit, Truth must be incorporated into one's mode of operation; thoughts and behaviors. Truth must be adhered to: 1) to be able to perceive and experience Spirit and 2) to manifest appropriate outcomes in thought, speech, behavior and materiality. If what one thinks and says are not true, the development of spiritual awareness will halt. Self-aggrandization is an example. As long as ego enhancement fantasies are spoken about and or fantasized in thought, the development of spiritual awareness will not take place. Truthfulness with ones own thoughts are prerequisite to the development of spiritual awareness. Even the truthfulness of what is said has a powerful influence on this development. If what is said is always truth, Truth will have an influence on what is said. If what is said is not truth, it will degenerate the consciousness of the sayer. Progress requires Truth. If one's mode of operation is founded in Truth, what one thinks and says will be Truth. This will make it possible for one's thoughts to consciously manifest into reality. The power of the Bodhisattva Spirit Warrior can then blossom.

Without the ability to discern Truth we cannot become aware of our limitations. Because the ego is so good at denial and rationalization, denial and rationalization become programed into our subconscious habits, influencing and determining our thoughts, behaviors and assessments. When this happens our thoughts and behaviors are based on illusion and the conclusions are irrational. The results are fear, stress and suffering. To overcome these habits we must develop the ability to apprehend Truth through the development of *objectivity* and its practice. Objectivity is the ability to perceive facts as they actually are; uninfluenced by previous conditionings, feelings or opinions. This ability must be self trained to make efficient progress.

Will - Personality purification requires the determination and discipline of a warrior. This is *will power*. The ego must be confronted, its belief system dissected and all its delusions exposed to the Sword of Truth. This is where the Spirit Warrior goes into battle. The ego refuses to give up its demons. The defeat of these demons depends on determination, patience, discipline, effort, self esteem and self confidence; which are all aspects of the Will. The Will is the key to motivate the sustained effort that is required to develop our spiritual awareness. The battle is won with the super exertion of the Will, of the Spirit Warrior.

Self-Examination is the starting point. All of our thoughts must be examined for appropriateness. All inappropriateness must be identified and the required changes made. All spiritual ignorance and inappropriate thoughts must be eliminated. This is the Process of Personality Purification. This process must continue until enlightenment is realized. Adversity offers the opportunity to use the tools of the Five Perfections and see the results that these tools can deliver. As results are obtained, confidence in the methods grow; which enhances the ability to obtain further results. The removal of all negativity cannot be accomplished without this Process of Personality Purification. It is the power of the Will that makes this possible. The Will is what drives the efficient application of the Process of Personality Purification. The Will is the key mental-spiritual attribute influencing the removal of negativity and the key to developing optimism.

The Spirit Warrior (continued)   Optimism, Gratitude and Forgiveness

Optimism and Gratitude

The Spirit Warrior must become perfect optimism. Optimism and Will are components of the magnetism that is required to attract into your life situations, circumstances and the mental and intuitional ability needed to accomplish our goals. The development of Gratitude will elicit Optimism and Joy. Once the consciousness becomes aware that: 1) the development of Love and compassion will remove all stress and suffering from the self and all others and 2) the opportunity to interact with creation is possible, unlimited and better than nonexistence, then the positive magnitude of this gift of life and existence, begins to appear. Meditate on this opportunity. See the depths of it. It will elicit Joy to be alive, Joy to interact with creation, Joy to incarnate on Earth and the opportunity to assist in bringing Joy to all sentient beings. The Gratitude that this realization elicits can bring the Willpower and the Optimism that is required to make the best out of our opportunity and achieve our goal.

Forgiveness of Others and the Self

Since the elimination of inappropriate thought habits and negativity are required for developing spiritual perception, all frustration must be replaced by perfect patience. Rude comments, foul language and negative thoughts must be eliminated. In order to maintain efficiency we must stay positive and optimistic even when we make mistakes. Guilt and animosity are negativity that must be identified, faced and removed from the personality. All transgressions that you feel were committed by and against you must be forgiven. You do not have to continue to interact with someone who has wronged you, but the wrong must be forgiven. The Process of Personality Purification is the application of choice. All thoughts and behavior are choices. If we choose to harbor guilt, animosity, negativity in any form, it will attract more stress and suffering. If we choose to stay positive and optimistic we will attract positive circumstances and Joy.

Guilt and animosity will create anxiety. Inappropriate thought habits and any negativity, will cause anxiety and symptoms of anxiety that will not only halt spiritual progress, but also cause emotional and physical stress that can cause chronic disease and possibly an early transition. Anxiety will deplete energy needed for: 1) health maintenance: mental, emotional and physical, 2) and the development of our spiritual awareness. Anxiety will deplete the energy required for mental focus, intellectual and intuitional ability (required for efficient self examination and spiritual perception). The removal of all negativity is part of the process of Personality Purification and will enhance the Process of Consciousness Energization. The Spirit Warrior must have the courage to face one's ego and forgive one's personality for the poor choices made and inappropriate behaviors committed.

As time goes by we change. Every thought we have changes us. As we go through the process of Personality Purification, we become a person that would not have made those previous mistakes. Eventually, we no longer become accountable. We become able to release ourselves from guilt. Our karmic debt begins to fade. Once the consciousness is completely operating from the perspective of Spirit, ones karmic debts will disappear. In order for the aspects of Spirit to perfectly manifest in the personality, all negativity must be removed. The Spirit warrior accepts this challenge. With perfect Love and Morality, Compassion and Charity, Determination and Patience, Discipline and Effort, Concentration and Meditation, the Spirit Warrior goes into battle and defeats the klesic demons.

Self Mastery

The Spirit Warrior must become a master of the self. Self Mastery is the ability to control one's thoughts and behaviors with Wisdom. It is required for mental focus in meditation. Any distraction from the mental focus required will easily halt the meditation process and the development of spiritual awareness. Negativity is probably the best example. Negativity will diminish the power of the Will and reduce the efficiency of thinking processes. It will cause anxiety and reduce energy levels. A manifestation of negativity of thought is the anticipation of negative outcomes of activities, events, situations and circumstances. It is caused by fear and the rationalization of feelings of self obsession, low self esteem, inability, and/or faineant. It is a habit of thought learned through conditioning and or traumatic experiences, often from childhood. This negativity is a product of our own thought. It does not exist in any part of Spirit. It has no Truth. Negativity has no power of its own. It is the energy of thought that gives negativity its power. But the undeveloped personality can and will make it manifest. Examples of negativity are excuses such as "I don't have enough energy" or "human beings are not capable of this" or "I am too tired" or "I don't know enough" etcetera. These thoughts can interfere with everything attempted. This negativity is a component of the worldly paradigm. Negativity of thought is a result of inadequate self-mastery. Negativity must be eliminated and self-mastery attained. This is done through the Process of Personality Purification and the practice of the Five Perfections.

The ability to efficiently stay on task, depends on self-mastery. Self-Mastery is driven by the power of the Will. Self mastery requires high energy levels, self training and a powerful Will. All maintenance and development regimens require self mastery. Examples are everything that we do: meditation, consciousness energization exercises, self examination, personality purification, health and hygiene regimens, nutrition, sleep habits, physical exercise regimens, activities of benevolence. Even the things that we do for fun are more enjoyable with self mastery.

Will

Will is the power of desire. The power of a desire is directly proportional to the value the consciousness gives it and the amount of energy available within the consciousness. The appropriateness of a desire is determined ultimately by the amount of Wisdom available within the consciousness (the lack of spiritual ignorance). Action upon a desire is determined by choice.

Will is the power, the psychic energy, that drives the action required to obtain what is desired. If the Will is not strong enough, the action required to obtain the desire cannot be accomplished. Operating from the worldly paradigm, from the time we are born into the world, our Will to survive is the strongest desire we have while we are existing in the flesh. When our natural worldly transition occurs, our Will to continue our sojourn becomes too weak.

Will is a component of creativity. Creativity involves our ability to recall pertinent information and assemble the information to solve problems. Efficiency depends on knowledge base, recall ability and thought processes. The higher the energy levels are, the easier it is to recall pertinent knowledge and to perform the required thought processes to solve problems. The use of intuition can dramatically increase the knowledge base and the performance of thought processes. High energy levels are required for the development of efficient recall ability, thought processing ability and intuition. The use of energy levels are controlled by the Will.

Psychological influences that degenerate the power of the Will are all the manifestations of the worldly paradigm: all ego defense mechanisms, negativity, low self esteem, low self confidence. The worldly paradigm is based on self centeredness. It is produced by the illusion of mortality. It results in an obsession with the self; an attachment. Self centeredness is a source of fear, anxiety, depression and negativity. Self centeredness is spiritual ignorance. This is a result of ignorance of what we really are; all powerful, immortal spiritual beings. Negativity is a habit of thought that is generated by this ignorance. It is the habit of thinking that we are vulnerable and incapable. It manifests in the thought or feeling of "I can't do that". Many imagined reasons are used: I am too dumb or too weak or too ugly or I can't control myself and many more. Another common form of negativity is to look for the faults of others. This is an attempt to overcome low self esteem, subconsciously telling the self that you are better than others in the comparison. The delusion that you are better than others causes stress and anxiety because it is a falsehood that you are trying to convince your self is true. The Truth is that we all are omnipotent, immortal spiritual beings. Because of self-centeredness, narcissistic behaviors will develop. This will cause social problems in your interactions with others, resulting in more stress, suffering and anxiety. These behaviors are a huge waste of time and energy. These thought habits must be removed. This is a major issue in the process of personality purification and consciousness energization. It is the power of the Will that drives positive psychological change; the elimination of negative thought habits and the elimination of spiritual ignorance. It is the power of the Will that drives the process of illumination.

Will (continued)

The influence of ones Will can operate at two levels: physically and metaphysically. Most obviously, the Will can be used to motivate oneself to do the things necessary for the maintenance of ones life: meditation, physical training, hygienic behaviors, nutrition, sleep habits, education, employment training, change employer, paint the house, plant the garden, etc.. Not so obviously, the Will can be used to metaphysically influence the situations and circumstances of ones life. With the application of one's Will and optimism, one can attract into ones life specific things and opportunities that are deemed beneficial: health, vitality, employment that will allow efficient service, specific environment in which to live, an appropriate spouse if needed, specific experiences, circumstances, Wisdom, Love, Joy, spiritual awareness, etcetera.

It is our Will that drives the action required for our enlightenment. In most cases the required Will seems almost superhuman. Will is a primary component of progress in the development of spiritual awareness and any endeavor. Will is the activating power behind self motivation (determination, discipline, effort). The power of the Will is directly proportional to the amount of energy available to the consciousness. The amount of energy available to the consciousness can be enhanced by: meditation, the application of the Will, focused concentration, the development and maintenance of physical health and vitality, the development and maintenance of mental health and vitality (personality purification, the removal of ignorance) and specific chi kung-pranayama exercises (consciousness energization). Meditation, San Zan, the Crane Breath and the Cobra Breath are consciousness energization exercises used within the Shaolin Tradition. The performance of any activity is enhanced with concentration. But efficient results in the training of the consciousness energization exercises is accomplished by the application of intensely focused attention. It is the application of a powerful Will that drives the intense concentration required for the efficient *metaphysical* transportation of chi-prana.

Will power is the key to the success of the Spirit Warrior. Will is the foundation of being. It is the power that motivates and continues our very existence. The Will is required to influence and manifest what we need in our environment. We use our willpower to direct and accomplish positive change as we work through the process of personality purification. Intuition is the only ability we have that will enable us to apprehend and experience Spirit. It is the key to the development of spiritual awareness. It is the energy levels within the consciousness that make intuition efficient enough to experience Spirit. It is the power of our Will that is required to raise the energy levels high enough to adequately activate and to direct our intuition, to accomplish this task. For the Spirit Warrior, the development of an indomitable Will is crucial. Our enlightenment will not occur without it.

The Spirit Warrior (continued)

Complete Spiritual Realization Is Inevitable

A Spirit Warrior is able to accept the challenge of the development of personal perfection and of any adversity that may arise. A Spirit Warrior knows that we are not given more than we can bare, and that if we can bare it, we can beat it. The Spirit Warrior has the determination and the tenacity to take the battle to its appropriate conclusion (Peace, Love, Wisdom, Joy).

Our habits of thought, determine our success or failure. If we think in self-defeating terms (negative thoughts) we will probably be defeated. If we think in positive, constructive and optimistic terms, incorporating the Five Perfections into the personality, we will succeed. The Spirit Warrior knows that his or her total spiritual realization is inevitable. And that the rewards are so great that the battle must be won as soon as possible. Because we are Spirit at the core of our beings, the Spirit Warrior knows that the strength, courage, and power of Spirit are available to all of us, at all times; even when we are experiencing the most difficult challenges.

The Spirit Warrior becomes fearless. The concept of failure or being a victim is not part of the consciousness of a Spirit Warrior. All negativity, insecurity, lack of confidence and all fear are removed from the personality. The Spirit Warrior trains sustained mental focus to enhance the efficiency of everything that is attempted. The klesic demons of self-centeredness, fear and ignorance, are defeated. All stress and suffering ends. It is then that the Spirit Warrior can become completely aware that we are immortal spiritual beings of Perfect Peace, Perfect Compassion, Perfect Love, Perfect Joy, Perfect Wisdom, Perfect Fearlessness, Perfect Illumination.

Orientation   The Summary of the Monk's Orientation   The Monk's Vow

The Monk's Vow makes an excellent summary for the subject of this chapter, Orientation to the Shaolin Monastic Tradition. This vow makes an accurate summation for what is required of a Shaolin Monk (a Spirit Warrior). This is the vow required for initiation into the Shaolin Sanga (monastic order).

The Vow of the Shaolin Monk

I will remove evil from my life with the Five Restraints:
    1) non violence   2) truthfulness   3) non stealing
                  4) sensual control   5) non possessiveness

I will cultivate virtue by incorporating into my life the Five Observances:
    1) purity   2) contentment   3) spiritual exercise
                  4) self examination/ purification   5) spiritual communion.

I will instill within my consciousness the Five Perfections:
    1) Perfect Compassion and Perfect Charity
    2) Perfect Love and Perfect Morality
    3) Perfect Determination and Perfect Patience
    4) Perfect Discipline and Perfect Effort
    5) Perfect Meditation and Perfect Illumination

I will assist in the liberation of all beings with the Five Daily Practices:
    1) service   2) self purification   3) spiritual study
                  4) meditation & prayer   5) surrender to God.

Through an exercise of my will and through the grace of God, I will bring into my life the complete awareness of Spirit in all its aspects:

    Love, Light, Compassion, Truth, Wisdom, Joy, Unity, Peace, and Bliss.

PART II

GOALS AND METHODS

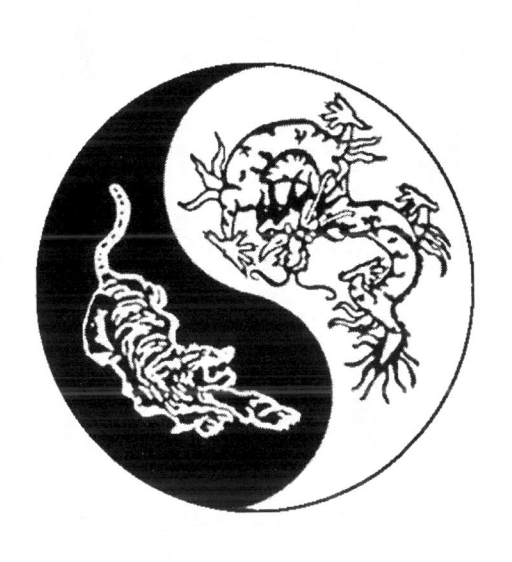

Goals and Methods of the Shaolin Tradition
The Shaolin Method for Personal Growth

The Goals of the Shaolin Tradition are perpetuated through compassion for all life, and to help bring an end to human suffering.

Some of the foundational teachings of this tradition are:
- that at the core of our beings we are Spirit,
- that suffering is rooted in the ignorance of the awareness that we are Spirit,
- that movement and meditation can be used to eliminate stress and end personal suffering by bringing a direct experience of Spirit, which culminates in the realization that we and everything, are Spirit,
- that this self realization will fill the experience of our existence with infinite eternal Joy and an awareness of Spirit in all its aspects, as we exist in Spirit, and participate in Creation, (Some aspects of Spirit are: Love, Light, Wisdom, Joy, Immortal.)
- that we assist in the positive evolution of Humanity for achieving these same goals.

The Shaolin Method for personal growth:
1) A personal commitment
2) Purification of the Personality
3) Energization of Consciousness
4) The 5 Perfections

1) A **personal commitment** to the goals of the Shaolin Tradition and its methods of achieving these goals must become a primary concern.

Living and life presuppose change. Change produces stress and without full knowledge of Reality, it sooner or later will produce suffering. Change in everything is inevitable; including change in your self. It is impossible to stay the same, either you change for the better or for the worse. This path is for those who decide they want to change for the better and solve the problem of stress and suffering with full knowledge of Reality.

The purpose of this training is holistic personal growth and to increase the quality of ones life (the Truth of ones life is never ending Cosmic Unity). A healthy body and mind assist in the development of spiritual awareness (developing a complete understanding and experience of Love, Truth, Wisdom and Joy). The body, mind and Spirit awareness are interrelated. A healthy body can more easily hold more energy. High levels of energy are required for mental acuity and stamina. A powerful mind is required to develop intuition sufficiently to use it to apprehend Spirit. This path is for those who recognize that life is a classroom where we are presented with lesson after lesson until we have learned each one in the process of perfection. Efficient progress in the development of these understandings demands active pursuit. Outstanding secondary benefits include higher energy levels, heightened awareness, developed mental capacities and self defense abilities. And as our spiritual awareness evolves we have a more positive influence on those around us and humanity.

2 - 2   Goals and Methods   The Shaolin Method for Personal Growth (continued)

2) Purification of the Personality The Shaolin term for Personality Purification, from its Sanskrit roots, is **Samasthana.** Self-purification of the personality is prerequisite to perceiving Truth and Reality (enlightenment).

One must match one's aspects of personality, to the aspects of Spirit in order to perceive and experience Truth and Spirit (Spirit is Reality).

This method requires that all thoughts be examined. Predominate thoughts and biases must be identified. All thoughts must be evaluated for appropriateness and self-directed change must occur if called for. All previous beliefs are to be re-examined for validity and re-examined again as more information is received and again, self-directed change must occur if called for. This process is repeated until perfection is attained.

Self-examination is required to expose yourself to yourself in the process of personality purification. In Self-Examination, one is expected to monitor one's self for any; negativity, fear, immorality, delusions, illusions, all intellectual limitations. One must become completely non-violent, truthful, non-stealing, non-possessive, and not do anything that will overly reduce energy levels. Narcissism, ignorance and fear must be completely eliminated.

The first step is identification of the inappropriate thought or behavior, through the process of Self-Examination.

Step two is the removal of the identified inappropriate thought or behavior. Removal is accomplished through a reaffirmation of the reason for the removal and an act of will with a conscious commitment to the removal.

Step three is continued monitoring of one's thoughts and behaviors for any repeated errors. As errors are identified repeat step two.

Affirmations and mantra can also be used to assist and accomplish the removal. The amount of energy required for the removal, is equal to the amount of energy the inappropriateness has within the personality.

When our own limitations are exposed to ourselves and identified, we can make the changes required to eliminate those limitations. Once adequate progress is made in this process of Self-Examination/Personality Purification, we can then efficiently develop the seven required abilities and manifest the Five Perfections through the Energization of Consciousness.

3) Energization of Consciousness

The energization of consciousness is required for the ability to perceive Spirit due to the poor intuitional ability of most humans. Intuition is the key to the direct experience of Spirit. The intuition requires large amounts of energy to work efficiently enough to do this. The Energization of Consciousness Methods are designed to perform this function. Some examples of these methods are: the Crane Breath, the Cobra Breath, the San Zan form and Meditation.

The efficient development of seven abilities are required and this development is also accomplished through the Energization of Consciousness. These seven abilities are: Intuition, Will, Concentration, Knowledge-Recall, Discernment, Objectivity, Self-Confidence. Aspects of these abilities can be developed through the process self examination/purification. Additional required development of these abilities can be accomplished through the practice of meditation and psycho-physical exercises (chi-kung/ pranayama, forms training). Once some development of these abilities is accomplished, then one can begin to manifest each of the Five Perfections.

Goals and Methods   The Shaolin Method for Personal Growth (continued)

4) **5 Perfections of the Shaolin Tradition**:
   1) Perfect Compassion develops Perfect Charity
   2) Perfect Love develops Perfect Morality
   3) Perfect Determination develops Perfect Patience
   4) Perfect Discipline develops Perfect Effort
   5) Perfect Meditation develops Enlightenment

The 5 Perfections of the Shaolin Tradition is a template of thought and behavior used to efficiently guide us through the process of developing the prerequisite abilities needed to experience Spirit. It is taught that perfection of the first virtue in each pair, develops the second virtue in the pair. The development of any pair enhances the potential of development of all the rest.

All five must be practiced with perfect non-attachment from the perspective of performer and beneficiary.

"Be ye therefore perfect, even as your Father which is heaven is perfect." - Jesus   Matthew 5: 48

Lao Tzu on Perfection
From the Tao Te Ching

To be crooked is to be perfected;
to be bent is to be straightened;
to be lowly is to be filled;
to be senile is to be renewed;
to be diminished is to be able to be receive;
to be increased is to be deluded.
Therefore the Holy Man embraces unity, and becomes the world's model.
He is not self-regarding, therefore he is cognizant.
He is not egotistic, therefore he is distinguished.
He is not boastful, therefore he has merit.
He is not conceited, therefore he is superior.
Inasmuch as he strives with none, there are none in the world able to strive with him.
The ancient maxim - 'To be crooked is to become perfected' - was it an idle word?
Verily, it includes the whole.

2-4 Goals and Methods   Positive Change   Self Discovery Learning   The Warning

Positive Change - Positive change requires understanding, knowledge, self examination and the self discipline required to make the changes that are called for.
Basically, there are two sources of knowledge:
    1) sources outside ourselves (i.e. what we are told, what we read)
    2) self-discovery, what we experience (intellect, inference, intuition).
Since what people say and write is prone to error (misjudgment or intentional deception) the only totally reliable source of understanding and knowledge is our own selves. Even then, to trust our own judgement requires much self-examination and self-training due to all the erroneous thought processes and behaviors we learn and accept as valid in our formative years. But a sincere, determined, disciplined effort will lead one to the goal of self discovery of Truth.

    Since this method of learning is scientific and based on first hand experience, the knowledge and wisdom gained is not "professed Belief". Professed belief is based on what is accepted as truth from sources outside yourself. The problem with professed belief is that you do not really know if it is true or not. This can cause high levels of anxiety and irrational behavior. The most horrific suffering of humanity has ben caused by egos defending a professed belief, e.g. almost all political and religious wars, the Christian Inquisitions, slavery, etc.

    The Mystic's Motto *"Assume Nothing"*.

Self Discovery Learning - Within the classic Shaolin Tradition "Answers are not given". Principles are presented for self analysis, testing and experimentation. Since this method is scientific, the Tao Chang and the world become a laboratory. Nothing is to be accepted as Truth until it is totally self tested; until Truth is experienced. This learning process facilitates the development of many of the mental abilities required for efficient progress toward our goal: direct perception and experience of Truth/Reality.

    Efficient self discovery learning requires prerequisite mental abilities. These are mental abilities required for reliable self-discovery to occur. The development of these abilities requires self-directed effort. These abilities are developed and enhanced through training in the methods presented by the Shaolin Tradition.

| **intuition** | self confidence | will | objectivity | discipline | determination |
| sincerity | discernment | memory | perseverance | integrity | concentration |

    Since this method of learning is scientific and based on first hand experience, the practitioner can develop the most efficient self-defense system possible; tailored for oneself. But here a warning is in order.

  - THE WARNING - Martial arts can be practiced to achieve the greatest good, but just like everything else in the universe, it does contain its opposite. Martial arts can also be practiced for the greatest evil. A dark side in the practice of martial arts, is the potential of violence inherent in it. Most personalities are attracted to the martial aspect of this activity and require an additional activity to balance themselves with the side of Light. It is the practice of meditation that the Shaolin Tradition uses to achieve this balance. The practice of martial arts can be a medium for personal development and a stepping stone to Self-Realization. But if it is practiced to enhance the ego and gain power over others, it will magnify ones delusion of separateness and move the practitioner farther from the experience of Love, Truth and an understanding and experience of the Unity of Humanity and the Unity of Spirit.

Goals and Methods — Spiritual Ignorance

Spiritual Ignorance - Sun Tzu, the author of the Art of War, wrote that you must know your enemy to efficiently defeat it. The enemy of one who walks the Path of the Five Perfections are the three klesic demons that exist within ones own consciousness: self-centeredness, ignorance, and fear. These demons must be identified and completely revealed to ones own consciousness to be efficiently eliminated. This is the purpose of the process of Self-Examination/Purification (the 2nd step in the Shaolin Goals and Methods).

When we are referring to ignorance, we are talking about spiritual ignorance. This ignorance is the source of all suffering. All insecurity is the result of ignorance. The result of insecurity is self-centeredness and fear. Even hate, possessiveness, aversion, all **attachments**, all non-organic mental illnesses and illogical habits are ways of coping with insecurity. When we eliminate ignorance we will have its opposite, Truth and Wisdom. With Truth and Wisdom we will have apprehended and experienced that we are immortal spiritual beings with all the aspects of Spirit: Immortality, Omnipotence, Omniscience, Omnipresence, Infinite Love, Compassion, Light, Truth, Wisdom, Joy, Peace, and Bliss. With this experience, even the biological drives become insignificant. With this knowledge and experience, the cause of all stress and suffering will be gone.

Ignorance is the cause of all suffering. This is why Loa Tzu wrote:
The highest attainment is to know non-knowledge (*1).
To regard ignorance as knowledge is a disease (*2).
Only by feeling the pain of this disease do we cease to be diseased.
The perfected man, because he knows the pain of it, is free from this disease (*3).
It is for this reason that he does not have it.

(*1) Non-knowledge is direct experience of Spirit through developed intuition. He calls it non-knowledge because the intellect is not involved.

(*2) Ignorance is the information we are told and read, the information our senses pick up and the conclusions we come to based on this information. Most often this information is coming from people who do not have full knowledge of what they are presenting or they are intentionally presenting false information for purposes of manipulation. The information coming from our senses is limited because it is incomplete. Our senses can not pick up information about the reality that exits beyond the worldly realm and the intellect is *very* prone to making mistakes due to its limited knowledge. Because this information and the conclusions we come to are based on information founded in ignorance, it will ultimately cause suffering; *it is a disease*.

(*3) Pain is the primary factor driving the motivation to solve the problem. Once one can identify and completely reveal this disease to oneself, we can take the steps required to over come it. Then we become *free from this disease*.

Lao Tzu said that we can make the changes necessary to eliminate ignorance " the disease"; that we can do this right within our own selves. We do this by reassessing and drawing accurate conclusions from our experiences using developed intellect and intuition.

Intellectual Limitations

Ignorance is the lack of Spiritual Awareness. With the defeat of ignorance, its opposite, Spiritual Wisdom develops. Wisdom will bring the awareness of the aspects of Spirit. The more the aspects of Spirit are incorporated into and become part of our consciousness, the more we are able to have direct experience, through our intuition, of Spirit. With developed Spiritual Awareness we can eliminate the disease of spiritual ignorance and the remaining demons will evaporate.

This is why Jesus said "Blessed are pure in heart, for they shall see God." - Jesus   Matthew 5: 8

God is a Spirit: and they that worship him must worship him in Spirit and in Truth.
Jesus - John 4: 24

Intellectual Limitations - a List of Ego Defense Mechanisms

These intellectual limitations must be identified and removed from the personality in the Process of Self Examination and the Purification of the Personality.

Ego defense mechanisms are intellectual limitations that, if used, must be exposed, identified and removed. All are an act of fear, an evasion of reality, an ignoring of Truth (ignorance). All cause stress and dramatically drain our energy. All are caused by insecurity. All are rooted in spiritual ignorance. Be fearless. Look into your inner world. Look at the root causes of your stress and suffering, your inappropriate thoughts and behavior and root them out. Take the sword of discernment, Truth and Wisdom to these demons and defeat them.

Rationalization - Attempting to prove that one's behavior is "rational" and justifiable and thus worthy of self and social approval.

Projection - Placing blame for difficulties upon others or attributing one's unethical desires to others.

Denial - Protecting the ego self from unpleasant reality by refusal to perceive or face it, often by escapist activities like getting "sick" or being preoccupied with other things.

Repression - Preventing painful or dangerous thoughts from entering the consciousness.

Reaction formation - Preventing dangerous desires from being expressed by exaggerating opposed attitudes and types of behavior and using them as barriers.

Identification - Increasing feelings of worth by identifying self with a person or institution of illustrious standing.

Fantasy - Gratification of frustrated desires in imaginary achievements.

Goals and Methods   Intellectual Limitations (continued)

Compensation - Covering up weakness by emphasizing a desirable trait or making up for frustration in one area by over gratification in another.

Introjection - Incorporation of external values and standards into the ego structure so the individual is not at their mercy as external threats.

Displacement - Discharging pent-up feelings, usually of hostility, on objects less dangerous than those which initially aroused the emotions.

Emotional insulation - Withdrawal into passivity to protect the ego self from hurt.

Isolation - Disconnecting the emotional component from hurtful situations or separating incompatible attitudes in logic tight compartments.

Regression - Retreating to an earlier developmental level involving less mature responses and usually a lower level of aspiration.

Sublimation - Gratification of frustrated sexual desires by substituting nonsexual activities.

Undoing - Atoning for and thus counteracting immoral desires or acts.

Sympathism - Striving to gain sympathy from others, there by bolstering feelings of self worth despite failures.

Acting-out - The reduction of the anxiety aroused by forbidden desires, by permitting their expression.

Further discussion:

A New Earth, Awakening to Your Life's Purpose: Eckhart Tolle *
2005, Plume   ISBN 978-0-452-28996-3

The Road Less Traveled: M. Scott Peck, M.D. *
1978, Simon & Schuster   ISBN 0-671-25067-1

"When the true nature of the universe and the relationship between it and one's essence of Being is known, and when one knows that lack of knowledge causes souls to forget their true Self and to suffer, one desires to be relieved of misfortune. Freedom from the bonds of ignorance then becomes the primary aim of life."   - Swami Sri Yukteswar

Meditation - Meditation is the foundation of the Shaolin Tradition. The main reason Bodhidarma was given the honor of being acknowledged as the 28th patriarch of Buddhism and being the 1st patriarch of the Chan Sect (Zen) is that he reinstated the requirement for the practice of meditation. In modern times, with the advent of the information age, more people are able to receive meditation instruction and receive the benefits of its practice. As meditation is becoming more popular, the more progressive spiritual traditions are beginning to incorporate it into their teachings. This is happening because more of humanity is beginning to feel a need to develop spiritual awareness and because meditation is the only efficient method of doing this.

Meditation is the very core of the methods taught within the Shaolin Tradition. All of the other methods and techniques that are taught, are practiced to develop and enhance meditation ability and its results. Even when meditation is the only method of developing spiritual awareness that is practiced, it will bring beneficial results. But when the Shaolin consciousness purification and energization methods are used in conjunction with meditation, complete spiritual realization can occur within the present lifetime.

Our five senses evolved to give us information about our material environment. Using these senses, it is impossible to acquire information that exists beyond this; which happens to be the vast majority of reality. The only sense that humanity has that can give us this kind of information is our sixth sense, intuition. Intuition can be used to acquire accurate information about anything, including and most importantly awareness of Spirit. The only efficient method of developing and using intuition for this purpose is through meditation. Meditation is the key to self knowledge, and the self realized experience of Spirit.

"Be *still* and know that I am God."   Psalms 46: 10

The Sign of the Experience of Spirit

Jesus said, "If they say to you, 'Where did you come from?', say to them,'We came from the Light, the place where the Light came into being on its own accord and established itself and became manifest through their image.' If they say to you, 'Is it you?' say, 'We are its children, and we are the elect of the Living Father.' If they ask you, 'What is the sign of your Father in you', say to them, 'It is *movement* and *stillness*.' "
             The Knostic Gospel of Thomas   Verse 50

"And ye shall know the Truth and the Truth shall make you free." - Jesus   John 8:32

Goals and Methods; Hsing

Hsing - Meditation in Movement (kata in Japanese, nata in Sanskrit, forms or sets in English)

The ancient mystic yogic warriors of India may have been the first to use ritualized martial movement to assist in the development of spiritual awareness. Their sanskrit term for these sets of movement was nata, hence the Japanese term kata. In the Shaolin Tradition, the practice of forms has aspects of both the Crane and Snake training methods. The Crane Methods (physical training) of forms practice acts as a preparation for the Snake Methods (spiritual training).

The practice of these sets has the potential of exposing our awareness to physical limitation that correlates to specific mental limitation; mental limitation that interferes with the development of spiritual awareness. The practice of these sets can be used as a technique for self examination, exposing flaws in our personalities that must be removed in the process of personality purification (removal of negativity, fear, self centeredness, anger, aggression, etc., all illusion and delusion). Personality purification must be performed to efficiently develop accurate perceptions of reality and spiritual awareness.

Some of these sets include movement, posture, and hand positions that are used to call our attention to spiritual concepts that assist in the development of spiritual awareness. These are called mudra. Through mudra, performance of the Temple Forms can become affirmations of one's life goals. Practice of the "Form of the Five Elements" will do this and help bring us into harmony with the forces of nature that influence the manifestation of creation; helping to clarify our awareness of reality and enabling us to perceive Truth more clearly.

The ability to perform martial movements spontaneously is developed through the practice of forms. The movements of the sequences are committed to memory and performed without any fore brain activity; without talking to yourself and telling yourself how to move. This is called Wu Hsin in Chinese (mu-shin in Japanese, dharana in Sanskrit) and translates as no-mindedness. It is sometimes referred to as the "Zen Mind" and described as "the ability to think without thinking". Wu Hsin is required for efficient self defense ability and any creative act (thought or movement). It is also a component of any intuitive experience and therefore a requirement for true meditation (concentration used to experience the Infinite). A scheduled routine of forms practice will develop Wu Hsin ability. The performance of forms in a state of Wu Hsin will allow the intuition to apprehend Truth. When the mind is in a state of Wu Hsin, the sthana (the ego, and all illusion and delusion) will drop away, the consciousness becomes exposed to reality. And when the intuition takes a look at it, one perceives the Ultimate Reality, Spirit. Form performance becomes meditation.

A scheduled routine of forms practice will develop mental abilities that can make one more efficient at what ever one does. These are some mental abilities exercised and developed through the practice of forms.

self confidence	effort	discipline	concentration
patience	memory enhancement	discernment	intuition
perseverance	will	determination	wu hsin

The mental abilities that are developed and trained through the practice of forms are prerequisite to the efficient development of spiritual awareness.

Goals and Methods: Chi Kung, Technique Drills, Martial Partner Practice

Chi Kung - This is the science involved in the use of Chi. Chi is the energy of Spirit. Chi is Spirit. It permeates all of creation and is what creation is made of. The ability to accumulate, conserve and transport Chi energy is Chi kung. Chi accumulation, balancing and distribution, controls: health, vitality, longevity, mental acuity, intuition and spiritual awareness. The Chi Kung methods used within the Shaolin Tradition are practiced to do all of these. The primary purpose being Consciousness Energization for the development of spiritual awareness. There is considerable overlap between forms training and Chi Kung since the practice of forms, to a great extent, incorporates the use of Chi Kung. San Zan, the Crane Breath, and the Cobra Breath are the primary Chi Kung methods used and are Bodhidarma's Brain and Marrow Washing Methods. When these methods are used with the Five Perfections Affirmations, they will assist in Personality Purification; training the personality purification and energization of consciousness simultaneously. The primary purpose of these methods is to energize the consciousness and develop the intuition to enhance the practice and results of Meditation.

Technique Drills are part of the Crane aspect of training. Within the presentation of the technique drills the principles of movement and fighting strategies are conferred. Learning the movements is an exercise in concentration. The practice of the movements develops many aspects of the mind-body relationship: coordination, timing, speed, flexibility, relaxation, balance, agility and stamina. This training develops confidence, self application, intensity of effort and the will; all of which are required for efficient development of spiritual awareness.

Basics are tedious, but;
    "The journey of a thousand miles begins with the first step."   - Lao Tzu

Martial Partner practice - This is a time for self analysis, testing and experimentation; of not only the martial aspects of practice but also the attitude, demeanor and motivations of yourself and your partner. Partner practice presents the opportunity to perceive *the other persons point of view*. Your partner practice should be a sharing experience. You are not to present techniques that are beyond your ability to deliver safely or your partners ability to respond to safely. Over zealousness is a manifestation of egotism and selfishness. Take the care required to keep from bruising yourself and your partner. Greater gains can be made when two people work together to learn. Instant feedback as ideas are examined and tested with a partner, speeds development of objectivity and discernment.

    Intuition can be enhanced and exercised during partner practice. Wu Hsin can be practiced and developed. These abilities can be turned toward an investigation of Reality to obtain a direct experience of the nature of Self and of the Infinite.

    "Look always, for the lesson in the situation."   - Shaolin Monk

    "The most skillful warriors are not warlike; the best fighters are not wrathful; the mightiest conquerors never strive; the greatest masters are ever lowly.
    This is the glory of non-strife; and the might of utilization; those equal heaven, they were the goal of the ancients."   - Lao Tsu

Goals and Methods — Sanshou and Personality Purification
The Detriment of Competition

Sanshou (Shiai in Japanese) Sanshou refers to detached fighting practice, within a formal match environment, used to develop spiritual awareness. But in the Shaolin Tradition this concept is *expanded to include all social encounters, situations and circumstances experienced in life*. The primary purpose of sanshou is personal growth; developing greater experience of Love, Truth, Wisdom and Joy. Development of these experiences demand active pursuit for efficient progress. Prerequisites to the development of these experiences are enhanced abilities of concentration, objectivity, will and intuition. Participation in sanshou, if properly motivated, can catalyze growth in these abilities.

Active pursuit of personal growth requires a period of self examination, then evaluation and corrective measures. The emotional nature of the sanshou presents an opportunity for latent attitudes and motivations (such as the desire to feel superior to others, gain power over others, fear, all the ego defense mechanisms, etc.) to express themselves and to expose them for Self-Examination and the Personality Purification Process.

The battleground is found within, not without. - Shaolin Monk

It is required that immediately after participation in each encounter that you sit quietly and contemplate the emotions, attitudes and motivations experienced before, during, and after the event. Then evaluate them for appropriateness. Any inappropriateness must be removed from the personality. This is done through an act of will; by making a firm commitment to the removal, and monitoring thoughts and behaviors for any repetition of the identified inappropriateness. Affirmations and mantra can also be used to assist and accomplish the removal. The amount of energy required for the removal, is equal to the amount of energy the inappropriateness has within the personality.

The attitude to strive for during sanshou is **detachment**. Motivation should be based on the results of the exercise and development of Love for All.

The Detriment of Competition

Modern main stream thought has made sanshou, partner practice and push hands practice competitive activities. This is a big mistake. Balance and harmony is impossible to obtain when the object of practice is to out-do the partner and win. The partner status is even lost. The other person becomes an opponent. Either the ego becomes enhanced and increases the delusion of separateness or the self esteem is diminished and the self confidence is reduced, which again increases the delusion of separateness. In either case an extreme is created, balance and harmony is lost. An advanced spiritual being who has experienced Unity awareness, such as a monk, cares for the well being of everyone. No one is an opponent. No one is an enemy. When competition becomes involved in the practice, the intended purpose of the training which is the direct experience of the principles and interaction of Spirit, completely disappears.

"When all desires that dwell in the heart cease, then the mortal becomes immortal, and obtains brahman."   - Upanishads

Goals and Methods — General Direction for Study
Advice from Master Sensei Eizo Onishi

Knowledge for which Ken Do Gaku members must strive:

You should know and understand the importance of the background of martial arts that is preserved in both literature and the physical training. Study and practice these two important aspects.

You must have confidence in yourself as a well educated person. Develop a good reading habit and be selective. Pursue your studies in the correct manner. You should follow them regularly and not become lazy or neglectful of them. Have the self care it takes to keep improving yourself.

<u>A **daily** schedule of study and training must be adhered to.</u> Once developed, the habit will assist in a sustained effort. Affirmations and autosuggestion may be helpful in maintaining enthusiasm and motivation.

Do not be concerned with victory or defeat. This makes a narrow minded and selfish person.

Train yourself to think with objectivity. It is not easy to overcome erroneous belief patterns and the tendency to rationalize, repress, etc.. It is impossible to come to know your Self if you cannot be honest with your own self.

You must learn to use your emotional nature with objectivity, for there is a limit to valuable knowledge that can be obtained thru objective thought alone. There is great truth to be gained from your feelings-intuition. (It is only through intuition that one can obtain direct experience of the Great Truth).

In order to practice an art (self expression) one must be creative. You must learn to use your emotional nature, for every creative act has an emotional component. True self expression can help bring self knowledge.

Look for and learn to perceive the many subtle social pressures that could be detrimental to your growth. Search within yourself to find the Truth. Do not blindly believe extrinsic sources.

Obtain a spirit of harmony and concordance with your fellow man, being courteous, respectful, and unselfish at all times. Come to understand the meaning of humility; experience the unity of humanity and Spirit.

Discover meditation; what it is, why it is done, how to do it. Develop a daily habit of meditation.

"Read not to contradict and refute, nor to believe and take for granted, nor to find fault and discourse, butto weigh and consider." - Lord Bacon

PART III

MEDITATION

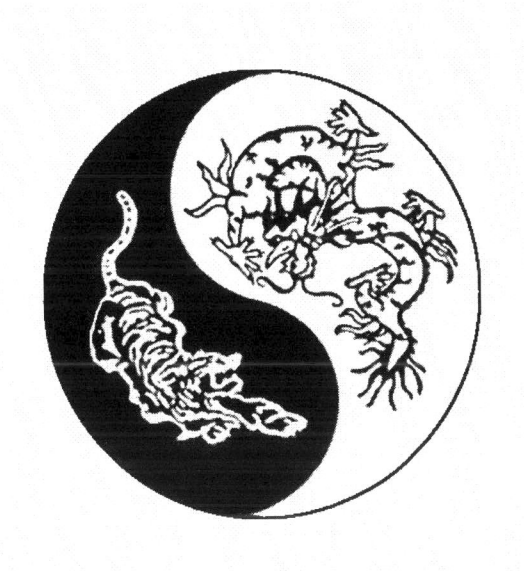

Meditation Information

3 - 1

Concentration Used to Know God

Goals of meditation are:
- to overcome the hardships that life can bring,
- to gain an accurate perception of reality (God),
- to discover for our own selves how direct communion with God can bring perfect bliss (heaven) in this life time,
- to learn how we can help others achieve this knowledge and experience;
    - and bring world peace and brotherhood to humanity.

Bodhidarma, the founder of the Shaolin Tradition, taught meditation, consciousness energization methods and martial arts for the purpose of developing spiritual awareness in the practitioners. Still, the primary goal of the Shaolin Tradition is the development of spiritual awareness. And even now, meditation is the primary method used to achieve this goal. Martial arts training, were then and still are secondary methods. Bodhidarma also used the martial medium to enhance the methods of the development of spiritual awareness that he taught. These techniques included methods of: personality purification, character development, intellectual development and the energization of consciousness. High levels of psychic energy are required for the intuitional ability needed to meditate effectively. He also taught advanced breathing techniques to adequately increase these energy levels. In addition to the purification of the personality, it is the energization of consciousness and the intuitional ability that results from these heightened energy levels, that is of primary importance to meditation success.

A goal of meditation is to gain an accurate perception of reality, which is the experience of Spirit and all its aspects. Meditation can be used to help bring this experience in this life time. This is **spiritual communion**. Through meditation we will learn how we can help others achieve this knowledge and experience; which will ultimately bring world peace and brotherhood to humanity. The most powerful positive influence we can have on humanity is to purify our own personality, energize our own consciousness and realize a direct experience of Spirit. This process is motivated by developed compassion. The positive influential power of the enlightened Bodhisattva is many, many, many times that of the unenlightened beings. There will come a time when the number of enlightened Bodhisattva will reach a critical mass where their influence will overwhelm the collective consciousness of humanity. This will enlighten the rest of humanity almost all at once, bringing Peace, Love, Joy, and Harmony to all those on Earth. Until then, which may not be in the too distant future, our enlightenment will come one at a time. Each one of us will martyr our little deluded self-consciousness for Universal Bliss. Obviously humanity is in need of more enlightened Bodhisattva.

Secondary benefits of meditation are: reduced stress, improved concentration, more ordered thought processes, enhanced intellectual skills, creativity is stimulated, the immune system and physiological processes are strengthened, biologic aging is slowed, regenerative energies are activated, intuition awakens, and appreciation for your life, the lives of others and all life is enhanced.

Meditation Information - continued

Our perception of reality is acquired through what our five senses are exposed to and the way we make sense out of the information our senses pick up. The problem is that our five senses can only detect limited and gross manifestations of reality within creation. The subtler manifestations that our five senses cannot detect, actually include the vast majority of reality. Modern science has only detected electrons and radio waves within the last century and there is so much more that it defies the imagination. We cannot even come close to an accurate perception of reality based on the information obtained from our five senses. It is important to take note here, the difference between learning by being told or reading about things and knowing through direct experience. Sources of information outside of direct experience are often limited and or incorrect. Even direct experience can be misleading when it is dependent on the five senses. Only developed intuition is infallible. The only tool we have that can enable us to detect and experience the rest of reality is our sixth sense, **intuition**. Meditation is the technique that can be used to efficiently develop and direct our intuition to obtain accurate knowledge and direct experience of Reality.

The organ of intuitional sight exists in man just behind the spot between the eyebrows. This spot is variously known as: the Spiritual Eye, the Single Eye, the Third Eye, the Ajna Chakra, the Star of Bethlehem, the Upper Tantien. A method of developing intuition, through meditation, is by directing the attention of the mind into this spot. The gentle raising of the gaze, with the eyes closed, will assist in directing the attention of the mind to this spot. This is sometimes called the **frontal gaze**. The attention focused into this spot will raise the energy levels in this area, thereby facilitating the development of intuition.

Spirit is omnipotent, omniscient and omnipresent. Spirit is creation, everything in it and everything beyond. Spirit is everything, even our selves. Spirit is reality itself. This can be known directly through intuition, by holding the attention of the mind on any aspect of Spirit, at the intuitional center (the spot between the eyebrows). Pick an aspect of Spirit that you feel an affinity with. Aspects of Spirit include: Divine Love, Light, Spirit, Truth, Wisdom, Joy, Peace, Bliss, Om. If you visualize the form of Christ you may intuitively experience His infinite Love and Divine Mercy or His consciousness of the Infinite Omnipresent Reality (Christ Consciousness). As the frontal gaze is held, allow your chosen aspect of Spirit to surround and permeate your consciousness. As your intuition kicks-in, your awareness of this aspect of Spirit will grow and develop into an awareness of Spirit in all its aspects and manifestations. Usually much practice is required.

Jesus said, "It is I who am the light which is above them all. It is I who am the All. From me did the All come forth, and unto me did the All extend. Split a piece of wood, and I am there. Lift up the stone, and you will find me there."
         The Knostic Gospel of Thomas   Verse 77

Jesus said this from the perspective of Spirit that exits at the core of all beings and all things.

Meditation Information - (continued)

Four Stages of Meditation

1. **Sitting and posture** is the first stage.
Face east as you practice meditation. Sit:
- with knees on floor, sitting on heels, in-steps on the floor (the Zen Meditation Posture)
- or with the legs crossed (full or half lotus),
- or on a chair, in the forward part of the chair with the back away from the back rest of the chair, feet flat on the floor

Place the hands palm up at the juncture between the thigh and abdomen.
   (a mudra of surrender of the little self)
Hold the spine straight but not strained (back, neck and head).
Keeping the spine straight, let go of all physical tension.
Hold the Frontal Gaze. Look steadily and with attention at the brow center.
   (With the eyes closed and do not strain).
Optionally, just before meditation, practice the crane or cobra breath
Then breath with the lower abdomen, not the chest. (Do not control the breath in any way)

2. **Inward turning** is the second stage; **sense withdrawal**.
Release all random thoughts, all worries and cares.
Hold the attention undivided.   Pay attention only to the presence of Spirit.
To hold the attention solely on this one activity will initially require considerable
   self directed effort.
When the attention wanders, gently bring it back time and again to the Frontal Gaze (into the Spiritual Eye) and one's chosen aspect of Spirit.
Sense withdrawal, includes detachment from:
- all thoughts (worries, cares and memories; conscious and subconscious)
- all physical sense stimuli (visual, tactile, auditory, olfactory, taste)
- all astral sensory stimuli (visions, clairvoyance, clairaudience, ect.)

Within the Spiritual Eye, only the outer ring of the Spiritual Eye is astral.
Practice brings proficiency.

3. **Actual meditation** - Undivided, focused attention on Spirit or an aspect of Spirit.

4. **Spiritual Communion** - Effortless, intuitive awareness of the Divine Self (the Great "One").

The Tao Te-ching   Lao Tzu   Chapter 47
   The world may be known without going out of doors.
   The heavenly way (Tao) may be seen without looking through the window.
   The further one goes the less one knows.
   Hence the Holy Man arrives without traveling;
       names without looking; accomplishes without action.

   Chapter 21   line 7 and 8
       How do I know the ways of all things at the beginning?
       I look inside myself and see what is within me.

Meditation Information - (continued)
Suggestions for Meditation,
Use of Affirmations and Mantra

Suggestions for Meditation

- Become God like; purify your consciousness observing the: Five Perfections, yamas and niyamas.
  Yamas are:
  non-violence, truthfulness, non-stealing, sensual control and non-possessiveness
  Niyamas are:
  purity, contentment, spiritual exercise, self study, and spiritual communion
- Do preliminary light exercise and or stretching.
  (Forms practice and or Hatha Yoga)
- Pray before and after meditation.
- Meditate in the same place when possible;
  this aids in conditioning for mental and physical stillness (stillness facilitates intuition)
  ideally in a place that is used solely for meditation, but this is not required.
- Try to meditate at least twice a day.
  The best times, in order, best first, are: dawn, dusk, midnight, noon
  Additional spare moments are helpful.
- Use a blanket to sit on and wrap your self in if it is too cool (use wool or silk).
- Affirmations or mantra may be used during the second and third stages of meditation, not the fourth stage.

"Blessed are the pure in heart; for they shall see God."
- Jesus   Matthew 5: 8

Use of Affirmations and Mantra

Affirmations are phrases and statements used to constructively alter and neutralize negative thoughts and thought patterns. They are delivered with positive energy commensurate with the negativity to be neutralized.
Examples are: In Perfect Peace I walk the path of the Five Perfections.
   I defeat the klesic demon of self centeredness and experience Spiritual Unity.

Mantra are phrases, words or syllables that refer to an aspect of Spirit and assist in mental focus that can lead the seeker into higher states of consciousness. Sanskrit mantra require specific pronunciation and usually require a teacher. Examples are: Omm, So Ham, Hung Sau. Other examples are: I am Love, I am Joy, or simply "God". These may be used in the second stage of meditation by quietly repeating the selected mantra, as each breath is exhaled.
   In the third stage of meditation it is repeated silently with each exhaled breath. And then "listened to", as each breath is exhaled.
   In the forth stage, the affirmation or mantra is allowed to drop away, and Spirit is experienced in the Divine Silence.

Meditation Information - (continued) Meditation Instructions

These instructions may be used when giving meditation instructions to a group.

Sit in a comfortable position.
Place the hands palm up at the juncture between the thigh and abdomen.
Hold the spine straight but not strained, shoulders back, chest box forward and jaw level.
With the eyes closed, gently raise the gaze toward the spot between the eye brows;
  and without any strain, gently hold this frontal gaze as we meditate.

Use the abdominal breath.
Breath only with the stomach not the chest or shoulders.
Breath naturally and slowly not trying to control the breath in any way.
Let the body relax,
  let go of all physical tension.
It is in physical and mental stillness that our awareness
  can efficiently perceive and experience the reality of Spirit.

Most importantly, fix the attention of the mind at the midspot between the eyebrows.
This is the center of intuition; the key to God perception.
Concentrate your attention here, with your awareness open to the presence of God.
If the attention should wander, gently bring it back, time and again to the frontal gaze.

A technique to help calm the mind is to watch the breath.
Do not try to control the breath in any way.
You will find that as you watch the body breathe,
  the breath will automatically become slower, deeper, and more rhythmic.
The mind and breath are inseparable, the condition of one will reflect the other.
So as the breathing becomes slower, the mind also will become more still.

In the stillness of peace,
  we rest in the awareness of the Divine Self within us
  and the omnipresence of the Great Spirit.

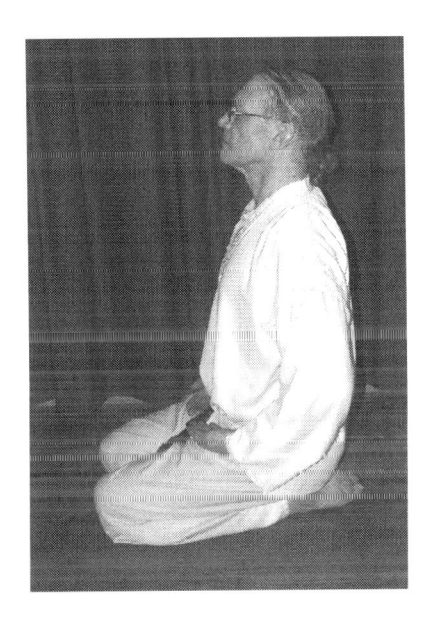

Meditation Preparation Techniques

Anuloma Viloma

This technique is usually performed as a preparation for meditation or chi kung practice. It is used to open the energy passageways (primarily the Ida and Pingala) and awaken Kundalini. Additionally, this technique will sooth and invigorate the nerves, clean the sinuses, improve digestion, and promote sound sleep.

Your regular meditation posture is assumed.
Back strait, body relaxed, jaw level, holding the frontal gaze
 and the mental attention focused in the Ajna Chakra.

Double exhale.
Using the Shiva Mudra, close off the right nostril.
Hold the breath for as long as it is comfortable.
Then, using the abdominal breath, slowly inhale through the left nostril.

Hold the breath for as long as it is comfortable, and slowly exhale through the left nostril.
Hold the breath for as long as it is comfortable and using the Shiva Mudra, close off the left
 nostril, using the abdominal breath, slowly inhale through the right nostril.
Hold the breath for as long as it is comfortable, and slowly exhale through the right nostril.
Change the nostril with the end of each exhale.

Alternate nostrils 18 times.

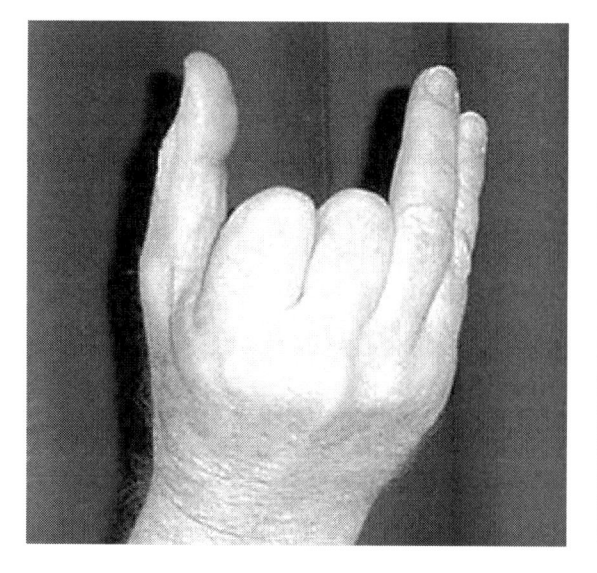

Shiva Mudra   Shiva Mudra Use

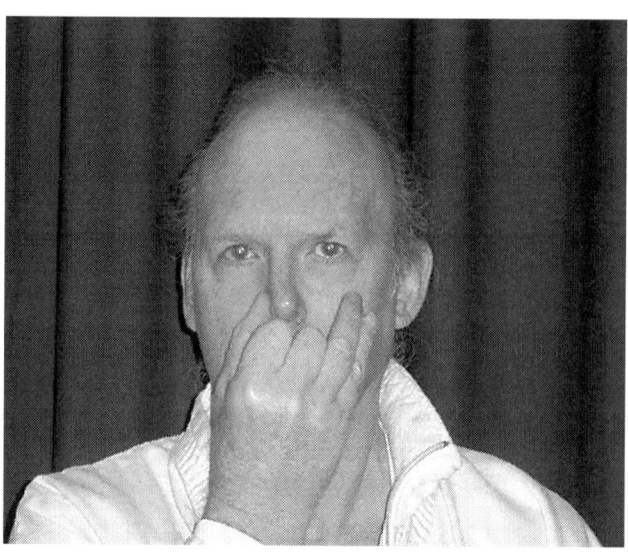

Meditation Preparation Techniques (continued)   The Bandhas

Bandhas   Also known as **The Gates of Brahman**

Bandas are techniques used to control blood and prana flow in the performance of asana and pranayama. The gates of Brahman are places along the cerebral-spinal path that narrow and slow pranic energy transportation. These bandhas are used to train pranayama methods to efficiently transport the pranic energy flow through these gates.

Mula Bandha   Root Lock

The mula bandha will block the energy from moving up the governing vessel and directs it up the cerebral-spinal path (the thrusting vessel). The mula bandha will force the transportation of prana upward from the mulahara chakra and swadhisthana chakra to the manapura chakra, thereby opening the first gate.

The mula bandha is performed by a simultaneous gentle contraction of the anal sphincter muscles and lift of the anus.

The mula bandha is usually performed in conjunction with the uddiyana pranayama, San Zan, crane breath, cobra breath. But it should be practiced until it becomes second nature.

Uddiyana Bandha   uddiyana means "flying up"

Uddiyana bandha is used to transport prana from the manapura chakra upward to the anahata and vishudha chakras. The manapura chakra is the launching pad for transporting prana to the anahata and vishudha chakras. This step is required to move from the worldly paradigm into the first true experience of spiritual perception. Adequate energy levels in the anahata and vishudha chakras will permit the first intuitive experience of Divine Universal Love and enhanced intellectual capacities. This is the opening of the second gate.

Uddiyana bandha is performed by pulling the abdomen inward and sucking the diaphragm up into the thoracic cavity.

The uddiyana bandha is used in the performance of the uddiyana pranayama.

Jalandhara Bandha   Throat Lock

The jalandhara bandha is used to stop blood pressure from rising too high in the head and brain when the breath is held too long and/or in the performance of inverted asanas. The rising blood pressure can cause capillaries in the head and brain to rupture. The throat lock and the third gate (cervical gate) will also limit the flow of prana to the ajna and sahasrara chakras.

The throat lock is performed by bending the head forward and placing the chin in the hollow of the neck.

Examples of the throat lock use are in the performance of the plow asana, shoulder stand asana, maha mudra and the uddiyana pranayama.

A variation of the jalandhara bandha is the **forward head drop**. The forward head drop is used to open the cervical gate for prana transportation into the ajna and sahasrara chakras. In a meditational asana, the head is allowed to fall forward to the jalandhara bandha position three to seven times. Then it is returned to the meditational posture for pranayama and/or meditation.

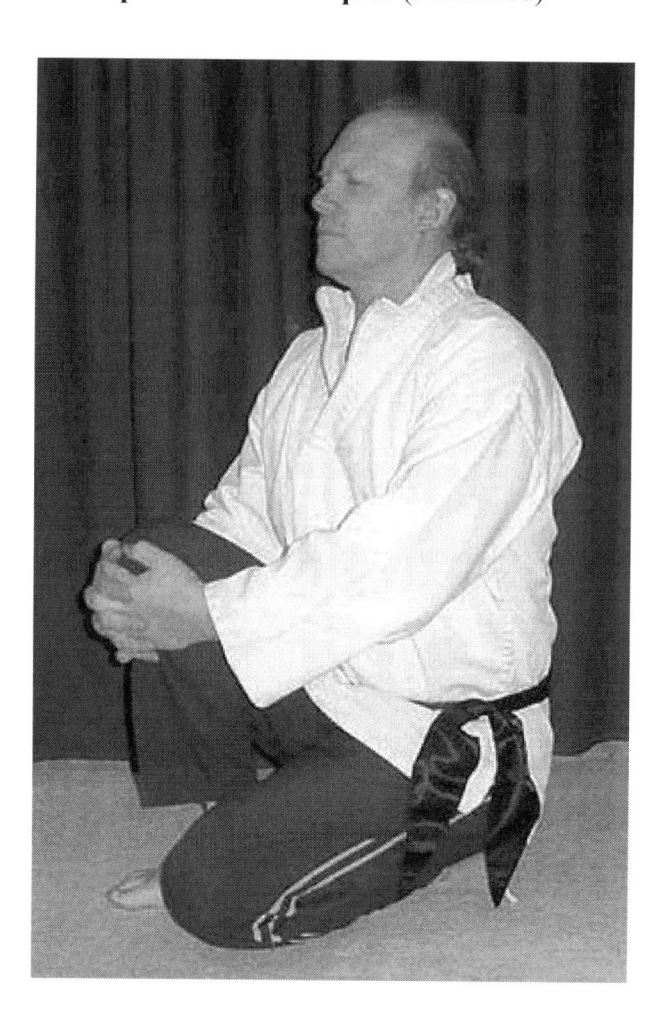

3 - 8 **Meditation Preparation Techniques** (continued)

Maha Mudra

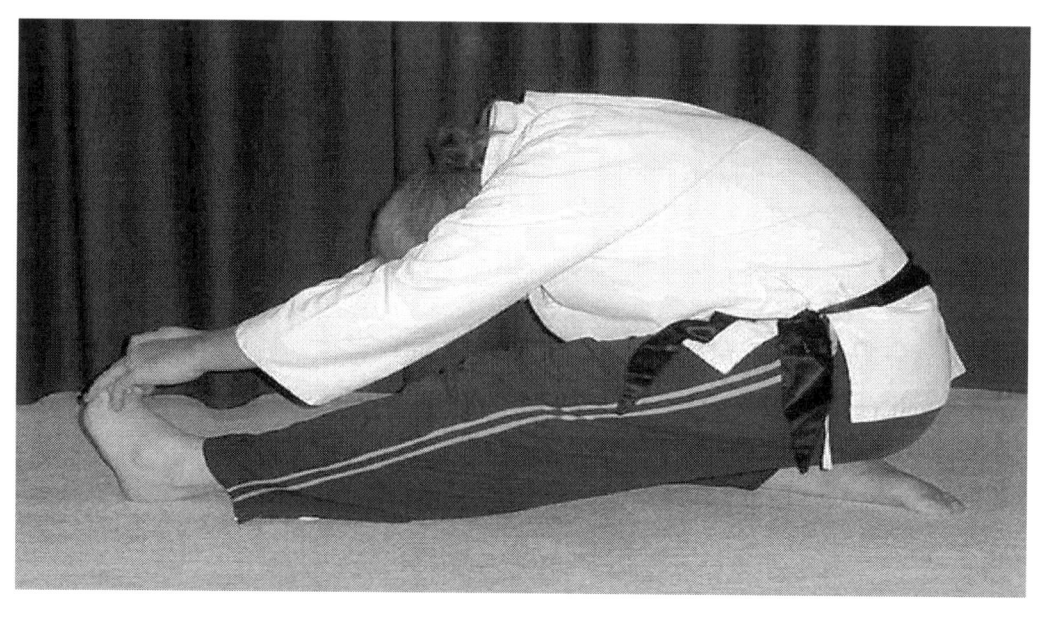

Meditation Preparation Techniques (continued)

Maha Mudra

This technique is usually performed as a preparation for meditation or chi kung practice. It is used to open the chakras and to prepare the Thrusting Vessel for energy transportation. Additionally, this technique will increase flexibility in the spine and legs, and make the energy in the body more available for transportation .

The Zen Meditation Posture is assumed.
This is also known as Vajrasan and Zazen.
Back strait, body relaxed, jaw level, holding the frontal gaze
  and the mental attention focused in the Ajna Chakra.

Start this technique by lifting and bending the left knee, entwining the fingers of both hands around the shin and pulling the leg into the chest.
Holding the back strait, body relaxed, jaw level, the frontal gaze,
  the mental attention focused in the Ajna Chakra, perform the double exhale, perform the root
  lock (anal sphincter contraction and lift), then inhale slowly (Crane or Cobra breath).
Hold the breath, perform the throat lock (chin to chest), straighten the knee, lean forward, and
  holding the ankle or foot with both hands, continue holding the breath, and the frontal gaze.
Hold the breath for twelve seconds mentally chanting OM with twelve heart beats.

The left leg is then returned to the chest by lifting and bending the left knee,
  entwining the fingers of both hands and pulling the leg back into the chest.
Holding the back strait, body relaxed, jaw level, the frontal gaze,
  the mental attention focused in the Ajna Chakra
The breath is now slowly exhaled.

Return to the Zen Posture and repeat the sequence with the right leg.

Then return to the Zen Posture and repeat the sequence with both legs together.

This completes one round of the Maha Mudra.

One to three rounds are performed before the Crane or Cobra Breath training.

3 - 10   Meditation Preparation Techniques: (continued)

Uddiyana Pranayama

This technique is usually performed as a preparation for meditation or chi kung practice. It is a thrusting vessel (Shushumna in Sanskrit) conditioning exercise for energy transportation through the thrusting vessel in preparation for Cobra Breath training. It is used to cause energy to rise up through the thrusting vessel and awaken the higher Chakras, increasing the experience of unselfish love and intellectual abilities. It will make sexual energy more available for intuitional purposes. The practice of this technique will enhance meditation practice. Additionally, this technique will tone the entire abdominal area, massaging virtually all the organs. It will squeeze blood, fluids and toxins out of the liver, spleen and pancreas, allowing fresh blood and fluids to revitalize these organs. It will reduce recall deterioration and increase longevity.

The Zen Meditation Posture is assumed.
This is also known as Vajrasan and Zazen.
Back strait, body relaxed, jaw level, holding the frontal gaze
  and the mental attention focused in the Ajna Chakra.

Perform the double exhale and hold the breath.
Gently contract the anal sphincter muscles and lift the anus (the root lock).
Perform the throat lock by bending the head forward
  and placing the chin in the hollow of the neck.
Place the hands on the thighs and lift the shoulders.
Pull the stomach in and suck the diaphragm up into the thoracic cavity (the uddiyana bandha).
Hold for twelve seconds mentally chanting OM with twelve heart beats.

Release and return to the Zen Posture with the hands on the thighs.
Slowly inhale while holding the Frontal Gaze.
This inhale can be performed in conjunction with the crane breath or cobra breath.

Meditate while the breathing returns to normal.
Then repeat two more times.

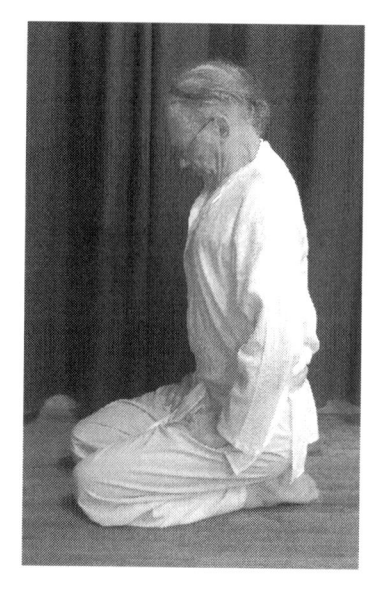

Meditation Preparation Techniques (continued)

Supta-vajrasan

This technique is usually performed as a preparation for meditation or chi kung practice. It is used to open the chakras and to prepare the Thrusting Vessel for energy transportation, aligning the vertebra and starting the transportation process by sending energy up the Thrusting Vessel. It strengthens the anal sphincter muscles and conditions the nerve plexus that works in conjunction with the base chakra to direct the energy up the Thrusting Vessel. Additionally, this technique will increase flexibility in the spine and hips, strengthen the abdomen and make the energy in the body more available for transportation. The ribs are strengthened, digestion and stomach imbalances are improved. Sciatica can be ameliorated and sometimes cured.

The Zen Meditation Posture is assumed.
This is also known as Vajrasan and Zazen.
Back strait, body relaxed, jaw level, holding the frontal gaze
  and the mental attention focused in the Ajna Chakra.

The hands are placed on and hold the back of the heals,
Gently contract the anal sphincter muscles and lift the anus (the root lock).
The elbows are straightened and the hips are pushed up and forward, causing a reverse back arch,
  as the head is dropped backward. (exhale as you rise into the posture)

Hold for twelve seconds mentally chanting OM with twelve beats of the heart.

Coming out, slowly and smoothly sit back down, then raise the head.

Meditate while the breathing returns to normal.
Then repeat two more times.

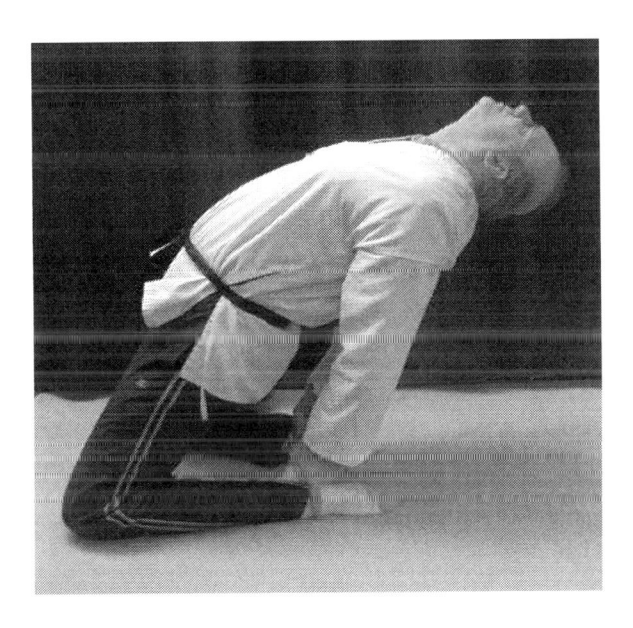

Meditation — Sense Withdrawal Techniques: (continued)

Wu Hsin Technique (Sanskrit is Neti Neti)

The meaning of the word "wu hsin" suggests "I am not thought". It is used in this meditation technique to achieve stillness of thought. Stillness of thought refers to not thinking with the use of words but allowing your awareness to open up to everything. As the intuition kicks-in, as you achieve the stillness, your awareness expands and you become aware of the Supreme Reality (the Ultimate Self, Spirit).

Your regular meditation posture is assumed.
Back strait, body relaxed, jaw level, holding the frontal gaze
 and the mental attention focused in the Upper Tan Tien (Ajna Chakra).

Begin to meditate, turn your attention inward into the spiritual eye.
The goal is to discover what you really are.
The method is to open up your awareness as you maintain perfect stillness.

The cue word used to develop the ability to maintain perfect stillness and to detach from internal
 and external stimuli is *Wu hsin*. Chant the word *Wu hsin* as each thought appears and return to
 the stillness. Practicing this technique while practicing stillness, will dramatically assist the
 development of the mental control required to achieve and maintain the stillness.

Practice of just five minutes a day can bring dramatic results.

This practice should continue until the goal is achieved.

"And when he was demanded of the Pharisees, when the kingdom of God should come, he answered them and said, The kingdom of God cometh not with observation: Neither shall they say, Lo here; or Lo there; for **behold**, the kingdom of God is **within you**."
                                             - Jesus   Luke 17:20-21

Jesus said, "If those who lead you say to you, 'See, the kingdom is in the sky,' then the birds of the sky will precede you. If they say to you, 'It is in the sea,' then the fish will precede you. Rather, the kingdom is inside of you, and it is outside of you. When you come to know yourselves, then you will become known, and you will realize that it is you who are the sons of the Living Father. But if you will not know yourselves you dwell in poverty and it is you who are that poverty."
                            The Gnostic Gospel of Thomas   Verse 3

Yoni Mudra

In order to turn inward enough to meditate efficiently one must be able to take control of the thoughts; to be able to focus the mind on one thing, without the mind wandering to something else. This includes the disengagement from thoughts that arise as the senses are stimulated.

This technique will assist in this detachment from the senses, but mental control and focus are still very much required. This technique will assist in developing the ability to see the light of the Spiritual Eye. This experience is auspicious because it is an indicator of substantial progress. It indicates that the ability to accumulate and transport substantial amounts of energy are being developed and that intuitional ability is being developed. Seeing the Spiritual Eye is the first step to the perception of the Colorless Five Pointed Star (the doorway to your direct experience of Spirit). The Spiritual Eye has been known by many names: the Third Eye, the Seat of the Soul, the Seat of Wisdom, the Star of Bethlehem, the Pentacle and many others. When it is completely seen it is made up of three lights: 1) a golden ring around 2) a blue disc and 3) a colorless star in the center. These are not visions or illusions. They are changeless, direct manifestations of Spirit that all adept meditators have seen throughout the history of humanity. This is the only phenomena, observable within creation, that is changeless. The ability to see this is characteristically a developmental process. Usually it is first seen as a hazy area of geometric designs. With continued, determined, disciplined practice it will begin to partially form and fade. The ability to concentrate and hold the attention is required to hold the complete awareness of the Spiritual Eye and to open the door. Generally, previous training and ability to transport energy into the Upper Tan Tien (Ajna Chakra) is required to obtain enough results to even recognize it when it is seen. With developed ability it will form with unmistakable brilliance.

"Knock, and the door shall be opened unto you." - Jesus   Matthew 7:7

Your regular meditation posture is assumed.
Back strait, body relaxed, jaw level, holding the frontal gaze
  and the mental attention focused in the Upper Tan Tien (Ajna Chakra).
The Yoni Mudra will work best after one or more rounds of the Cobra Breath are performed.

The senses are closed off with the finger tips.
The thumbs are placed over the tragus (the flap over the hole into the ear)
  and pushed to close the ear opening.
The index fingers are placed over the bottom of the eye lids and used to hold the eye lids shut and
  the eye balls in position for the Frontal Gaze. It is important to use only enough pressure to
  accomplish this.
The middle fingers close the nostrils.
The ring fingers are placed on top of the lips and the little fingers are placed underneath the lips.
  These fingers are used to close the mouth when the breath is held.
Optionally, a table or adjustable rack can be used to assist in holding the arms up.

Meditation   **Sense Withdrawal Techniques: Yoni Mudra** - continued

Double exhale and use the Cobra Breath to draw the energy into the Upper Tan Tien.
The chakra mantras can be used in this process.
When the inhale is complete, hold the breath and continue to mentally chant Om as the Frontal Gaze is held, as long as comfort allows.
If you have transported enough energy into the Upper Tan Tien and if your concentration is sufficiently focused, the Spiritual Eye will begin to form as the Frontal Gaze is held.
When the breath can no longer be held with comfort, exhale with the Cobra Breath back to the base chakra and repeat the process.

This process is performed three times. Each time turning deeper inward.
When the third breath is exhaled, perform the inhale of one Cobra Breath drawing the energy into the Upper Tan Tien again.
Continue to meditate in the stillness, holding the awareness of the Spiritual Eye as long as possible.

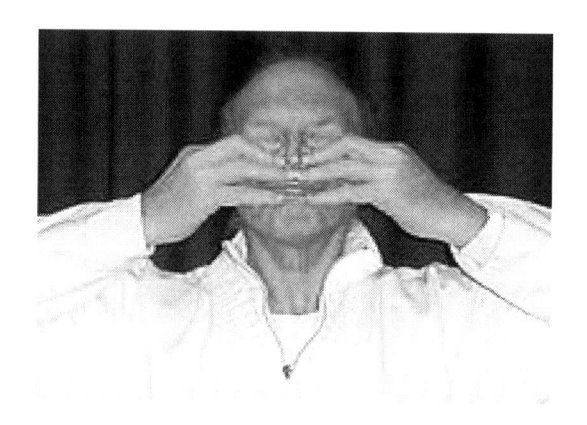

Yoni Mudra finger placement

"The light of the body is the eye: if therefore thine eye be single,* thy whole body shall be full of light." - Jesus Mat. 6: 22

* the single eye - is the point between the eye brows, the intuitional center; the seat of spiritual vision in man.

Soo Hum Meditation Technique

This meditation is usually performed after chi kung/pranayama practice.
It can be performed either before, during or after regular meditation practice.
It does not matter what time it is practiced, what matters is that you practice it.
What matters is that it is practiced daily, at the same time and the same place.
The subconscious mind is comfortable with habit and habit builds efficiency.
The Soo Hum Meditation Technique will release the awareness from body consciousness, develop mental control, raise energy levels and will move the awareness into the meditational state.

Your regular meditation posture is assumed.
Hold the back straight, body relaxed, jaw level.
Hold the frontal gaze and the mental attention focused in the Upper Tan Tien (Ajna Chakra).

Without any conscious control, breath abdominally.
Watch the body breath completely on its own.
Waiting for the inhale to occur all by itself, mentally chant Soo.
And when the exhale comes mentally chant Hum.
With each naturally occurring inhale, mentally chant Soo and with each naturally occurring, exhale mentally chant Hum.
The experience of Divine Peace will grow.

As the body continues to relax, the breath will naturally become slower and a natural pause will occur between inhales and exhales. As the pauses occur, allow yourself to experience the perfect stillness that exists within the pauses.
The perfect stillness will allow the experience of bodily detachment; the conscious awareness of existence without the body and attunement with the illuminative state.

Once the Stillness and Peace become constant the chant can be released and you can remain in the meditation as long as you want.

The perfect peace and stillness that will continue to grow as you get deeper into the technique, will allow energy to flow into your being and will make it possible to enhance the experience.

The breath ties us to self identification with the body. In the intervals between breaths we can gain release from this tie, achieving what is known as the "breathless state".

The Omm Meditation

This meditation is usually performed after chi kung and or pranayama practice.
It can be performed either before, during, or after regular meditation practice.

Your regular meditation posture is assumed.
Back strait, body relaxed, jaw level, holding the frontal gaze
  and the mental attention focused in the Upper Tan Tien (Ajna Chakra).

The meditation begins by chanting the mantra Omm;
  not loudly, with a medium-low pitch, with each exhaled breath.
The exhale begins with OOOO and the last fifth of the exhale with M. OOOOOOOOMM

Do not just listen to the Omm sound, fill your consciousness with it,
  allow your consciousness to be surrounded and permeated with it.
Allow yourself to become the Omm.

After a while, as you continue the chant with each exhaled breath, begin to chant the Omm mantra a little quieter.
Then quieter with each exhaled breath and quieter until you are whispering it.
Then mentally with each exhaled breath.
Then just "listen" to the chant with each exhaled breath.

As your intuition kicks in and you become one with the Omm, you will slip into satori.
The inner sound of OM naturally arises into the awareness.
Since Omm is the first expression of Spirit, as it brings creation into manifestation,
  this experience will eventually bring an awareness of Spirit in all its aspects.

"These things saith the Amen,
        the faithful and true witness,
                the beginning of the creation of God;"
                                                    Rev 3:14

The origin of the word Amen is the ancient Hebrew word for Aum; which is another word used for Om. When Aum or Om replaces Amen in this verse, the meaning becomes clear.

Chakra Light Meditation

    This technique is usually performed after regular meditation practice. Your regular meditation posture is assumed: back strait, body relaxed, jaw level, holding the frontal gaze and the mental attention focused in the Upper Tan Tien (Ajna Chakra). Begin by moving your awareness to the base chakra, totally experiencing the *energy* and *light* of the chakra, then lift it up through the Thrusting Vessel to the next chakra. This is continued by moving the *energy* and *light* upward through each chakra. As it rises, the energy and light becomes more subtle and more intense.

    Place your awareness into the center of the base chakra, the **Mulahara**. Experience yourself as yellow light and its yellow rays of light emanating from this chakra. Fill your awareness with this light and *feel* yourself as this light and energy.
Optionally affirm: *I exist in Joy as an entity of Spirit. I prosper in the abundance of Spirit.*

    Next move your awareness into the center of the sacral chakra, the **Swadhisthana**. Experience yourself as white light and its white rays of light emanating from this chakra. Fill your awareness with this light and *feel* yourself as this light and energy.
Optionally affirm: *I exist as Peace in the awareness of Spirit.*
    In Bliss I experience the infinite manifestations of Spirit.

    Continue moving your awareness upward into the center of the abdominal chakra, **Manapura**. Experience yourself as red light and its red rays of light emanating from this chakra. Fill your awareness with this light and *feel* yourself as this light and energy.
Optionally affirm: *I exist as the omnipotent energy of Spirit. I express compassionate Vitality.*

    Continue moving your awareness upward into the center of the heart chakra, **Anahata**. Experience yourself as smoky green-blue light and its rays of light emanating from this chakra. Fill your awareness with this light and *feel* yourself as this light and energy.
Optionally affirm: *I exist as Divine Love, with humility and compassion I serve Humanity.*

    Continue moving your awareness upward into the center of the throat chakra, **Vishudha**. Experience yourself as sparkling sea blue light and its rays of light emanating from this chakra. Fill your awareness with this light and *feel* yourself as this light and energy.
Optionally affirm: *I exist as omniscient Wisdom, incarnated as a Bodhisattva.*

    Continue moving your awareness upward into the center of the brow chakra, **Ajna**. Experience yourself as snow white light and its rays of light emanating from this chakra. Fill your awareness with this light and *feel* yourself as this light and energy.
Optionally affirm: *I exist as Omnipresent Awareness. Divine Unity is flowing through me.*

    Continue moving your awareness upward into the center of the crown chakra, **Sahasrara**. Experience yourself as colorless white light and its rays of light emanating from this chakra. Fill your awareness with this light and *feel* yourself as this light and energy
Optionally affirm: *I exist as the omnipresent brilliance of the spiritual Light. I am Spirit.*
    I am Infinite Light, Love, Wisdom and Joy.

    After reaching the Thousand Petaled Lotus (the crown chakra), return to the base chakra and reascend 3 to 108 times.

    As the meditation deepens, the consciousness expands into the Light of Spirit.

From **The Song Celestial**
    Also known as the **Bhagavad Gita**
    which is a part of the **Mahabharata.**

An excerpt from Chapter VI Religion by Self-Restraint.
    Krishna is speaking.

        The sovereign soul
Of him who lives self--governed and at peace
Is centered in itself, taking alike
Pleasure and pain; heat, cold; glory and shame.
He is the Yogi, he is Yukta, glad
With joy of light and truth-dwelling apart
Upon a peak, with senses subjugate
Whereto the clod, the rock, the glistening gold
Show all as one. By this sign is he known
Being of equal grace to comrades, friends,
Chance-comers, strangers, lovers, enemies,
Aliens and kinsmen--loving all alike,
Evil or good.
           Sequestered should he sit,
Steadfastly meditating, solitary,
His thoughts controlled, his passions laid away.
Quit of belongings. In a fair, still spot
Having his fixed abode--not too much raised,
Nor yet too low--let him abide, his goods
A cloth, a deerskin, and the Kusa-grass.
There, setting hard his mind upon The One,
Restraining heart and senses, silent, calm,
Let him accomplish yoga, and achieve
Pureness of soul, holding immovable
Body and neck and head, his gaze absorbed
Upon his nose-end*, rapt from all around,
Tranquil in spirit, free of fear, intent
Upon his Brahmacharya vow, devout,
Musing on Me, lost in the thought of Me.
That Yogin, so devoted, so controlled,
Comes the peace beyond--My peace, the peace
Of high Nirvana!

* Swami Sri Yukteswar explained "origin of the nose" is the point between the eyebrows: the seat of spiritual vision.

PART IV

**CHI KUNG
TRAINING METHODS**

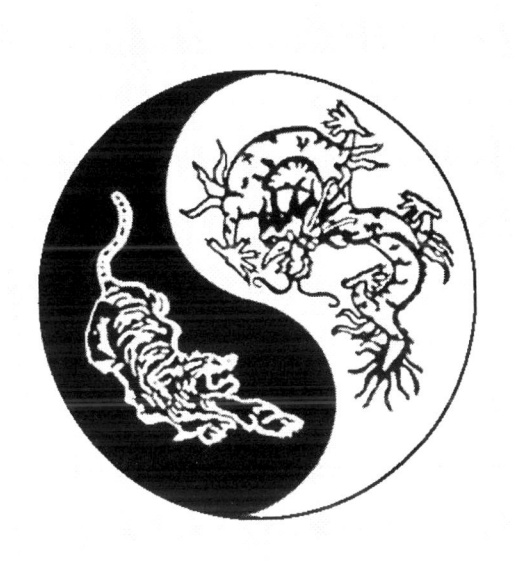

Chi Kung Training Methods

Chi Introduction

The movement of Spirit is responsible for the manifestation of creation. Spirit, beyond creation, exists in perfect stillness and in Chinese is called *Wu Chi*. The vibration of Spirit is called *Tai Chi* and is what brings all matter and energy into existence. The energy that manifests from this vibration is *chi*. Chi permeates all of creation and is what it is made of. The oscillations of the vibration have what is termed a positive side (yang) and a negative side (yin). Depending on these vibrations, all matter and energy, even circumstances, can have a yin or yang polarity. Some gross examples of this polarity are found in the opposites of day and night, summer and winter, male and female. According to chi theory, nothing can be completely yin or yang; there is always something of the opposite present in everything. Day is never so bright that it blinds us, or so hot we burn to death. Night is never so dark that we totally cannot see, or so cold we freeze to death. This polarity will influence the behavior of all matter and energy. In chi kung applications, to achieve optimum health, the energy (chi) in the body requires high levels and a balance of the yin and yang polarities. To raise awareness of Spirit, intuitional ability must be developed. Intuitional ability is developed primarily through meditation and consciousness energization exercises. Consciousness energization exercises are chi kung applications used to raises energy levels available to the consciousness. The culmination of these efforts are used to produce a personal experience of the Spirit.

Internal Energy versus External Energy

The concepts of internal energy and external energy refer to the use of two different energy sources. External energy originates solely from the brute strength of muscular power. Internal energy is derived through the use of chi (called *chi* in Chinese, or *prana* in the yogic tradition). Chi strength influences the vitality levels in the body. The San Zan form has traditionally been practiced to build this internal energy and the vitality levels. Methods, such as this, that are used to accumulate and transport chi are called *chi kung* in Chinese or *pranayama* in the yogic tradition of India. The ability to use internal energy usually requires years of intense effort, and is much more powerful and versatile than external energy. It can be used for martial applications, but more importantly it is used for physical, mental and spiritual healing and development of the self and others.

Chi Accumulation, Balancing and Transportation

The San Zan form is performed while holding considerable tension in the body (about 70%). Research in the west has shown that this type of isometric exercise will develop physical strength. At the beginner level, San Zan is an example of *wai dan chi kung*, which are the methods used to accumulate chi in localized areas of the body. The other type of chi kung is called *nei dan chi kung* which is used to accumulate and transport chi through the chi vessels and meridians of the body. The chi vessels and meridians make up the chi circulatory system. Nei dan chi kung can be used in advanced practice of San Zan. Other examples of nei dan chi kung are the crane breath and cobra breath. Chi accumulation and transportation is required for energizing the upper tan tien to the levels necessary for spiritual realization. Chi accumulation, balancing and distribution, will influence: health, vitality, longevity, mental acuity, intuitional ability and spiritual awareness.

The Rule of No Extremes

The requirement of balance in the yin and yang polarities has resulted in the Rule of No Extremes. This rule requires us to never take thoughts or behaviors into an extreme. Simply stated, <u>do not take anything to an extreme</u>. Eating is a good example. If we eat too much we will get fat and experience all the negative symptoms this will elicit. This is an extreme of eating too much. If we do not eat enough we will get weak and eventually die, the extreme of eating too little. To maintain optimum health we must eat the appropriate amounts of food and nutrients. If we train our bodies too hard we will injure our selves damaging muscle, tendons, and joints, which will slow and easily halt our progress. If we do not train hard enough we will not achieve the required results. The basic example of the extremes of procrastination and fanaticism are both stressful. Both will cause energy loss and the deterioration of health. To stay healthy and effective our activity must stay balanced. The delivery of marital movement requires a balance of tension and relaxation. Too much tension in the muscles as the movement is delivered will slow the movement down. Too much relaxation and the movement will not have the required power. This rule is internalized in the practice of T'ai Chi. In T'ai Chi it becomes obvious in the rules of movement, as no appendage is ever fully extended or fully retracted, the weight shifts are not more than 70% and 30% to one leg or the other, movement is performed with no more tension than with what is required, which allows relaxation in movement.

The Super Human Abilities of an Enlightened Master

The Rule of No Extremes operates within the realm of creation but not in the realm of Spirit. All of creation and everything in it is a manifestation of Spirit and is maintained by it. Creation is unimaginably huge, but there is an end to it. Within Creation there are rules that control its operation, maintenance and evolution. Spirit exists limitlessly beyond creation. When we allow our consciousness to merge with Spirit we can rise above the rules that operate within creation. We can even assist in its operation and maintenance. This is what makes the super human abilities of an Enlightened Master possible.

The Five Primary Training Methods

Our being and consciousness exist in three sheaths: a physical body, an astral body, and a causal body. Each body is a less gross manifestation of the previous body and vibrates at a higher rate. The causal body is the first manifestation of Spirit and the least gross and highest vibrational rate. The chakras are organs of the astral body. The chakra system is a series of energy centers situated along the cerebral-spinal axis. These energy centers influence the personality in a developmental progression to maturity; from self absorption to selflessness. The energy of Spirit (prana/chi) that animates us and gives us life, enters our beings at the chandra chakra (the feminine side of the ajna chakra) near the medulla and descends through the chakra system to the mulahara chakra (the center at the base of the spine). The energy then rises back up through the centers, but pools at the center of the maturity level that our personality has achieved. Within the Shaolin Monastic Tradition, there are five primary methods of purifying our consciousness and raising the level of this energy pooling. These primary methods are used to produce higher levels of maturity and spiritual awareness. The first two methods are preparatory for the more advanced and esoteric training. These preparatory methods are known as the Shaolin Crane System and come from Bodhidarma's Muscle and Tendon Changing Methods. The esoteric methods are known as the Shaolin Snake System and come from Bodhidarma's Marrow and Brain Washing Methods.

1) The first method is the process of **Self Examination/Personality Purification or Purification of Consciousness**. Spiritual awareness is dependant on the development of the aspects of Spirit within the personality. *One must match one's aspects of personality, to the aspects of Spirit, in order to perceive and experience Spirit.* The techniques within this first method can eliminate negative thought patterns and behaviors that can waste large amounts of energy. This energy waste is caused by illusions and delusions that produce the immature personality orientations. These illogical belief patterns produce the suffering within ourselves and within humanity causing further huge energy loss. Efficient mediation cannot occur with the loss of this energy.

2) The second method (The Shaolin Crane System of Methods) involves preparing the physical body for the Snake Training. This second method aims at hygiene, health, strength, stamina, and flexibility, etc. (salt water cleanse, stretching, nutrition, forms training, etc.). A healthy physical body dramatically enhances the methods practiced within the Snake Training.

3) The third method is the first of the esoteric methods of the Shaolin Snake System of Methods. It involves the practice of energy-control techniques. Illogical belief patterns and karmic influences are recorded and are acted upon within our chakra system. The removal of this negativity is accomplished with the pranayamic/chi kung methods (cobra breath, chakra energization and chakra purification techniques).

4) The development of our intuitional ability is the fourth primary method. Intuition is our only sense that can give us information and experience of Spirit. It is the key to spiritual realization. The development of spiritual awareness depends on the development of our intuition. And *the development of intuition depends on high levels of psychic energy* (chi/prana). Chi kung/pranayamic techniques (the crane and cobra breath, San Zan, etc.), in conjunction with meditation, are used within the Shaolin Monastic Tradition to develop our intuition for this purpose. This **Consciousness Energization Process** is used to dramatically enhance meditation ability.

The Five Primary Training Methods (continued)

5) Meditation is the fifth method which includes sense-withdrawal, concentration, meditation, and results in enlightenment.

Development within any one of these methods enhances the potential for development of the others. Training begins with the first two methods. With initiation, all the methods are trained simultaneously.

Chakra Developmental Personality Maturity Construct and Chakra Personality Orientation Characteristics

Mulahara - The Base Chakra   Survival   First Dimensional Consciousness

The personality orientation of this chakra is concerned with the requirements to preserve one's own life; satisfying the basic requirements for survival: food, shelter, clothing. Within this orientation one will do what ever it takes to secure the necessities for bodily survival and what ever is perceived to be what is needed. There is a predisposition to restlessness, insecurity, fear and material interests. The moral belief is that since the self is the only thing that has value, whatever can be taken by force for the needs of the self is justifiable. Obedience can be acquired from a powerful authority. Fear of punishment can determine behavior and attitudes. One will not consider the needs of another person unless it will benefit oneself to do so. The moral belief is in the survival of the most fit, and might makes is right.

Muladhara Chakra Information: Astrological influence; Saturn   Color; yellow   Mantra; lam
Element; earth   Sound; C and like a bumble bee   Asana: posterior stretch, butterfly
Affirmation: *I exist in Joy as an entity of Spirit.*
  I prosper in the abundance of Spirit.

Swadhisthana - The Second Chakra   Sex, Reproduction and Creativity
  Second Dimensional Consciousness

Within the personality orientation of this chakra, one recognizes that the immediate family is a necessary component of one's survival. Because of this, one recognizes that the security of the immediate family has substantial value. Concern develops for providing assistance for the needs of the parents and siblings. One begins to see the self as part of the family and the family as part of the self. There is a predisposition to sexual obsession, fantasy, insecurity, confusion, fear and material interests. The moral belief is that since the immediate family is the only thing that has real value, whatever can be taken by force for the family is justifiable. For the family, theft from others outside the family and even murder could be justifiable. Might is right. This Chakra is the seat of the yin polarized chi; this is the Shaolin Tiger energy, in yoga it is called Shakti.

Swadhisthana Chakra Information: Astrological influence; Jupiter   Color; white
Element; water   Asana: boat, prone spinal twist   Mantra; vam   Sound: D and flute
Affirmation: *I exist as Peace in the awareness of Spirit.*
  In Bliss I experience its infinite manifestations.

Chi Kung Training Methods
Chakra Developmental Personality Maturity Construct
and Chakra Personality Orientation Characteristics - (continued)

Manapura - The Third Chakra   The Body's Battery
                               Power   Third Dimensional Consciousness

    Within this personality orientation one recognizes that the extended family, the clan, tribe and or nation is a necessary component of one's survival and recognizes that the security that this larger group provides has primary value. Concern develops for providing assistance for the needs of the this group. One begins to see the self as part of this group and this group as part of the self. The focus becomes the preservation of the society and not just obeying as in the previous orientations. There is a predisposition to behaving according to social norms. Insecurity, fear and self esteem issues cause stress and can drive behaviors. The moral belief is that since the nation has primary value, whatever is perceived to be required to provide for the security of the nation can be taken by force (resources, lands, lives, etc.). This is why wars are fought. These people believe that the laws of the land are what make things right. These people believe that no matter what the situation or circumstances that are involved in the infraction of a law, the unlawful act is wrong.

    At the present time, the vast majority of humanity operates within this personality orientation.

Manipura Chakra Information: Astrological influence; Mars   Color; red   Element; fire   Mantra; ram   Sound; E and harp   Asana: locust, bridge, fish
Affirmation: *I exist as the omnipotent energy of Spirit.*
                       I express compassionate Vitality.

Anahata - The Fourth Chakra
         The Source of Our Awareness of Universal Unconditional Love
                       Feeling Love   Forth Dimensional Consciousness

    In the first three chakra personality orientations, behavior is motivated by fear; of stress, of suffering and feelings of insecurity concerning the self and those that help provide security for the self. Due to the developing intuition, thoughts and behavior begin to be motivated by Love and Compassion. Within this personality orientation, humanity becomes ones primary concern. Concern develops for providing assistance and for the needs of this group. Unity awareness begins as one begins to see the self as part of humanity. The moral belief is that what is right is determined by universal ethical principles that apply to all people and all nations based on Love and concern for all of humanity, individually and as a whole. These principles take precedence over any given social law. This orientation requires the use of some developed intuition since there is no physical evidence that the loss or condition of people that one does not even know, will have any effect on one. This orientation represents the first step into a spiritual perspective. Worldly motivations of ego-enhancement, fear and insecurity; superiority, competition, power over others, etc., will start to drop away. The intellectual abilities and personal integrity become more developed and the Five Perfections begin to manifest.

Anahata Chakra Information: Astrological influence; Venus   Color; smokey blue-green   Element; air   Asana; seated spinal twist   Mantra; yam   Sound; F and gong or bell
Affirmation: *I exist as Divine Love. With selflessness and Joy, I serve Humanity.*

Chi Kung Training Methods
Chakra Developmental Personality Maturity Construct and
Chakra Personality Orientation Characteristics - (continued)

Vishudha- The Fifth Chakra
 The Source of Our Awareness of Cosmic Understanding
  Expressing Love   Fifth Dimensional Consciousness

Within this personality orientation all of life has become ones primary concern. Concern develops for providing assistance for the needs of the this group. One begins to see the self as part of all life. There is an attraction to developing knowledge. Powers of intelligence and intuition enable perception deep into reality. The moral belief is that what is right is determined by universal ethical principles that apply to all people and nations based on Love and concern for all life, individually and as a whole. While in this orientation one must continue to use effort to remain true to the Bodhisattva vow. Awareness becomes soul conscious. As the awareness evolves, Divine Love and Compassion motivates compassionate behavior that will assist others in the development of their spiritual awareness. Each of these advanced orientations require the use of more intuition than the one that precedes it.

Vishuddha Chakra Information: Astrological influence; Mercury   Color; sparkling sea-blue
Element; ether   Asana: plow, shoulder stand   Mantra; ham   Sound; G and ocean's roar
Affirmation: *I exist as Omniscient Wisdom, incarnated as a Bodhisattva*

Ajna - The Sixth Chakra
 The source of our enhanced intuition and the doorway into spiritual perception.
  Experience of Spiritual Unity   Sixth Dimensional Consciousness

Within this personality orientation all of creation has become ones primary concern. Concern develops for providing assistance for the needs of the this group. One begins to see the self as part of creation. The moral belief is that what is right is determined by universal ethical principles that apply to everything in Creation, based on Love and concern for all of creation. This chakra is the seat of consciousness and the director of energy transportation. Seeing the Spiritual Eye in this chakra, is the first step to the perception of the Colorless Five Pointed Star (the doorway to your direct experience of Spirit). When it is completely seen, it is made up of three lights: a golden ring around a purple disc and a colorless star in the center. Awareness becomes God Conscious as one begins to experience clairvoyance, omniscients, omnipresents,. Each advanced orientation requires the use of more intuition than the one that precedes it.

This Chakra is the Upper Tan Tien, the seat of the yang polarized chi; the Shaolin Dragon energy. It is the interaction of the Tiger and the Dragon energies, (Sanskrit, Shakti and Shiva) in the union of the required amounts of these polarized energies, that catalyzes the reaction that produces the expansion of consciousness.

Ajna Chakra Information: The Ajna Chakra is the omniscient, omnipresent spiritual eye.
Chandra Chakra: is the feminine half of the Ajna Chakra, located at the medulla.
Astrological influence; Ajna Chakra, Sun - Chandra Chakra, Moon   Color; snow-white
Sound and Mantra; A and Omm   Asana: cobra, camel

Since the influence of this chakra comes from the soul, which is a direct manifestation of Spirit, no element is associated with this chakra.
Affirmation: *I exist as Omnipresent Awareness. Divine Unity is flowing through me.*

Chi Kung Training Methods
Chakra Developmental Personality Maturity Construct and
Chakra Personality Orientation Characteristics - (continued)

Sahasrara - The Seventh Chakra   The Source of Our Experience of Spirit
              Experience of spiritual Divinity   Seventh Dimensional Consciousness

Within this personality orientation one recognizes that Spirit is the only reality and the worldly personality disappears. It is recognized that the personality was a fabrication of consciousness that it used to cope with the world. One begins to see the self and everything as Spirit, existing within Creation and beyond. The moral belief is that what is right is determined by universal ethical principles that apply to all people and all nations, based on a perception of reality from a perspective of Spirit. This orientation requires totally developed intuition as one experiences omniscients, omnipresents, omnipotents, and all the aspects of Spirit (Love, Light, Compassion, Truth, Wisdom, Joy, Peace, Bliss, etc.). This experience will free us from all stress and suffering.

Sahasrara Chakra Information: Sometimes called *The Thousand Petalled-Lotus*.
Since the influence of this chakra is pure Spirit and beyond creation, no planet, color or element is associated with it. Sound and Mantra: B and bam   Asana: savasan, or any meditative posture
Affirmation: *I exist as the omnipresent brilliance of the spiritual Light.*
              I am Spirit. I am infinite Light, Love, Wisdom, Joy.

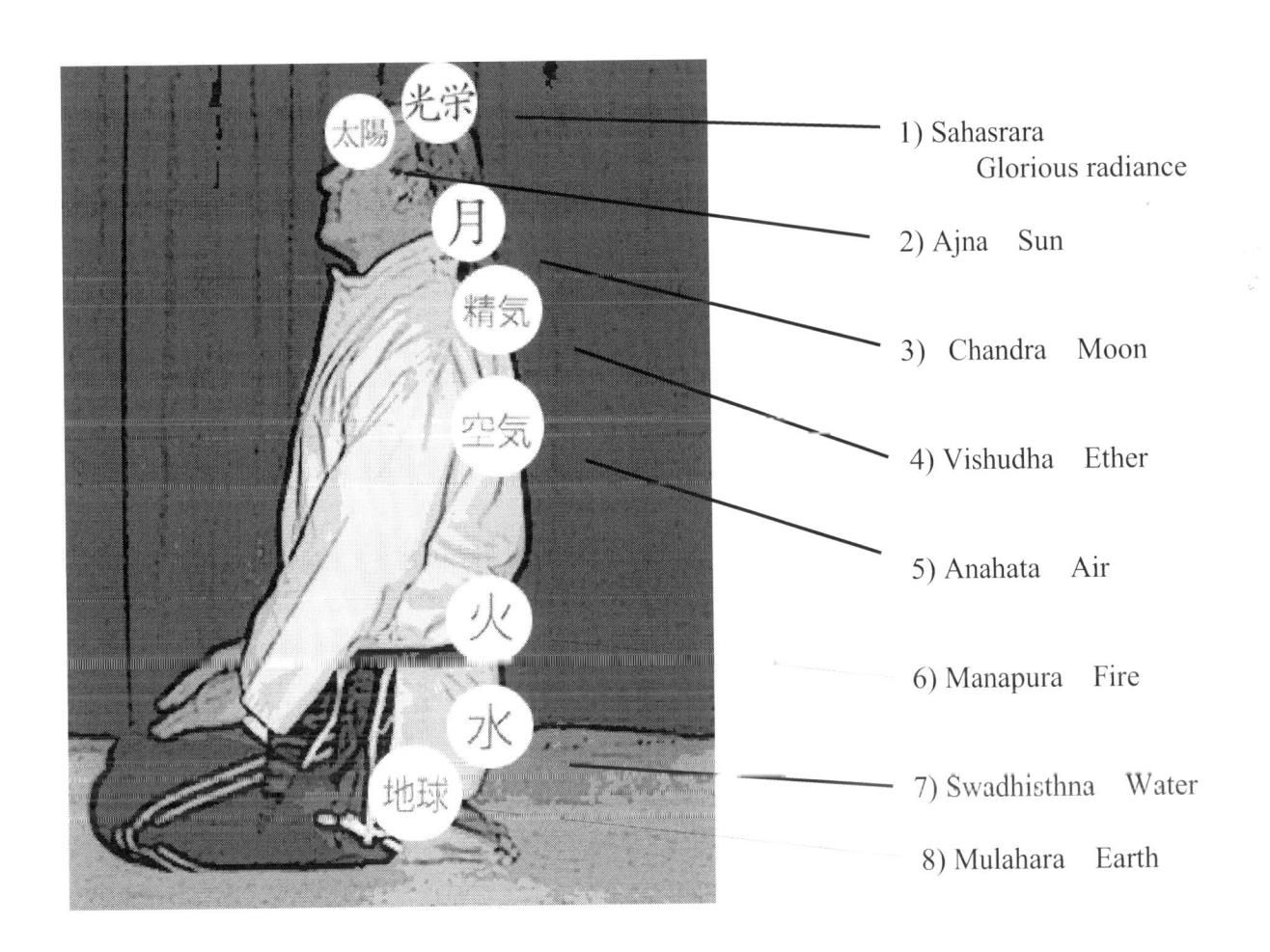

1) Sahasrara
    Glorious radiance
2) Ajna   Sun
3) Chandra   Moon
4) Vishudha   Ether
5) Anahata   Air
6) Manapura   Fire
7) Swadhisthna   Water
8) Mulahara   Earth

Spiritual Birth

The Swadhisthana Chakra is the seat of the yin polarized chi in our astral bodies; this is the Shaolin Tiger energy. In Buddhist and Hindu Mysticism this yin energy is called Shakti, the feminine kundalini energy. Shakti is the consort of Shiva. In Hebrew and Christian Mysticism, this is the energy of Eve. Eve is the consort of Adam.

The Upper Tan Tien is the Ajna Chakra, the seat of the yang polarized chi; the Shaolin Dragon energy. In Buddhist and Hindu Mysticism this yang energy is called Shiva, the masculine kundalini energy. In Hebrew and Christian Mysticism, this is the energy of Adam.

At this micro level within creation, it is the interaction of the Tiger and the Dragon, the union of the required amounts of these polarized energies, that catalyzes the reaction that produces the expansion of consciousness. At the macro level, it is the interaction of these cosmic energies that manifest all of creation and in this process the holy sound of Omm is produced.

It is in the union of these two energies in the Spiritual Eye (Upper Tan Tien, Ajna Chakra) that creates the spiritual orgasm that results in the birth of the awareness of the Great Self. The fetus is nourished with the energy work in the lower Tan Tien and whose birth is prepared for in the Thrusting Vessel in the cerebral-spinal axis. The spinal cord, medulla and brain look like a cobra snake; hence, the Path of the Snake and the Cobra Breath. The fetus is given birth through the tunnel in the Spiritual Eye (the birth canal) as the cosmic sound of Omm is heard. And is then released into the Light of Spirit as it passes through the Star. The soul, freed of all its attachments in Creation, spreads its wings of brilliant light and flies into the experience of the awareness of God.

The Story of Spiritual Birth in Genesis; the origin of the Bridal Chamber Sacrament

This story, in Genesis, was most probably told by someone who did not have full understanding of the story's meaning. The story-teller may have embellished the story so he could make some sense out of it. Since he seems to recommend against the use of the subject of the story, it is possible that he could be intentionally misleading the reader for a manipulative purpose. The reason could be: just plain ignorance and fear, possibly to insure that the seeker is prepared or it could be to retain control of the reader. After the results of this method are produced, no possible worldly control can be effected. Look what Jesus did. In either case, the mystic can still see the original meaning.

Chi Kung Training Methods   The Story of Spiritual Birth in Genesis - (continued)

Ge 2:7 *And the LORD God formed man of the dust of the ground, and breathed into his nostrils the breath of life; and man became a living soul.*

The *breath of life* is the energy and consciousness of God, chi/prana, that animates our being. Concentration, will, and the *breath* are used to do the energy work involved in this method to energize the consciousness and efficiently develop spiritual awareness.

Ge 2:17 *But the tree of knowledge of good and evil, thou shalt not eat of it: for in the day that thou eatest thereof thou shalt surely die.*

God is speaking here. Why would knowledge of good and evil cause death? In Ge 3:5 the snake assures Eve that eating the fruit will not cause death. In Ge 3:22 God says that eating the fruit will bring the awareness of immortality, which seems to contradict this statement. Does God lie? Maybe God is talking about the death of the immature ego consciousness which will usher in the birth of Christ Consciousness. It could be the story-teller does not have complete knowledge of the subject. Possibly the intention is to create fear in the unprepared so they will not consider the use of the method (see page 7 - 11 Cobra Breath Warning).

Ge 3:1 *Now the serpent was more subtle than any beast of the field which the LORD God had made.*

The serpent represents the cerebral spinal path that Eve walks to achieve union with Adam. This path runs from the sacrum to the pituitary gland. It is the spinal cord, medulla, and brain; and looks like a cobra snake. The snake is used repeatedly in various mythologies to make this reference. This serpent path is very subtle, it is the astral energy channel called the Thrusting Vessel, (the Shushumna in Sanskrit). This path runs up the center of the spinal cord to the Spiritual Eye.

The union with Adam occurs in the Upper Tan Tien. In Sanskrit it is called the Ajna Chakra. Jesus called it the Bridal Chamber. Jesus alludes to it in some of his parables in the New Testament. In the Gnostic Gospel of Philip this method of developing spiritual awareness is called the Sacrament of the Bridal Chamber.

Ge 3:4 *And the serpent said unto the woman, Ye shall not surely die:*
Ge 3:5 *For God doth know that in the day ye eat thereof, then your eyes shall be opened, and ye shall be as gods, knowing good and evil.*

When the Spiritual Eye completely opens, the intuition will allow the experience of the self as an aspect of God, in all of God's aspects (immortality, omnipresence, omniscience, omnipotence, compassion, Love, Light, Truth, Wisdom, Joy, Peace, Bliss, this will remove all stress and suffering) *and ye will* surely *be as gods.*

Jesus answered them, Is it not written in your law, I said, "Ye are gods"? Jesus - John 10:34

Ge 3:6 *And when the woman saw that the tree of life was good for food, and that it was pleasant to the eyes, and a tree to be desired to make one wise.*

The Tree of Life is the Chakra system in the astral body, that can be used to nourish and energize the consciousness to a level where the awareness expands into God Consciousness. The Tree of Life is a major subject in the Kabala, the Hebrew book of mysticism. This book explains that the Tree of Life is the Chakra System and how it can be used to develop spiritual awareness. The phrases *"pleasant to the eyes"* and *"to make one wise"* are a little bit of an understatement.

4 - 10   Chi Kung Training Methods   The Story of Spiritual Birth in Genesis - (continued)

Ge 3:7 *And the eyes of them both were opened.*
This is saying that the method works.

Ge 3:22 *And the LORD God said, Behold, the man is become as one of us, to know good and evil: and now, lest he put forth his hand, and take also of the tree of life, and eat, and live for ever:*
"*To know good and evil*" is another reference to Wisdom. "*And live for ever*" is another reference to immortality.

Ge 3:24 *So he drove out the man; and he placed at the east of the garden of Eden Cherubims, and a flaming sword which turned every way, to keep the way of the tree of life.*
The east is the direction we gaze when we meditate and practice this method. "*The Cherubims and the flaming sword*" appear to be placed to block the path to Self Realization. They are referring to the difficulty in obtaining the knowledge, the practice and the results of the method. Bodhidarma said that the initiated monk had to stare at the wall for nine years before obtaining the results. *To keep the way of the Tree of Life*, the Cherubims represent the difficulty in walking the Path of the Five Perfections; the psychological demons that must be defeated in the process of personality purification and the energization of consciousness. The flaming sword refers to the Spiritual Eye. Although the Spiritual Eye is very subtle when initially perceived, when the yellow disc forms it is very defined and glows. But when the Spiritual Light is first seen, it seems blinding. The Spiritual Light is accessed through the Spiritual Eye. Jesus calls it the Single Eye. This is where the masculine and feminine energies (Adam and Eve, Shiva and Shakti, the Tiger and the Dragon) achieve union and give birth to the Consciousness of Christ. This is the Bridal Chamber Sacrament that Jesus taught his disciples.

"For as the lightning, that lighteneth out of the one part under heaven,
             shineth unto the other part under heaven;
                   so shall also the Son of Man be in his day."
                   - Jesus   Luke 17: 24

"God is Light and in him is no darkness at all."   - I John 1: 5

"The light of the body is the eye:
       if therefore thine eye be single,
             thy whole body shall be full of light."
                   - Jesus Mat. 6: 22

Chi Kung Training Methods   Chakra Correlation Within the Lord's Prayer

Prayer Phrase	Chakra Correlate	Prayer Phrase
Our Father,	Sahasrara	Forever and ever.
Who art in heaven,	Ajna	And the Glory,
Hallowed be thy name.	Vishudha	The Power,
Thy kingdom come,	Anahata	For thine is the Kingdom,
Thy will be done,	Manipura	And lead us not into temptation But deliver us from evil.
On Earth as it is in heaven.	Swadhisthana	As we forgive those who trespass against us.
Give us this day our daily bread	Mulahara	And forgive us our trespasses,

    The meaning of each phrase actually correlates to the meaning and maturity level within each chakra. This is no coincidence. How could it be, given the complexity of the correlation? Jesus obviously used the Lord's Prayer to teach the performance of the esoteric methods of the Process of Purification and Energization of Consciousness to his disciples. Apparently, Jesus taught The Lord's Prayer as part of the Sacrament of the Bridal Chamber.

    The first method is to say the prayer and move the mental awareness to the energy center of the associated phrase as each phrase is recited; first column of phrases down and second column up.

Chakra Correlation of the phrases within The Lord's Prayer

Sahasrara   *"Our Father"*   *"Forever and ever"*
    Within the orientation of this chakra the consciousness is experiencing its self as Spirit.
   "Our Father" refers to Spirit, the source of Reality. "Forever and ever" refers to the infinite and immortal nature of Spirit.

Chakra Correlation of the phrases within The Lord's Prayer - (continued)

Ajna   *"Who art in Heaven,"*   *"And the Glory"*

Within the orientation of this chakra, the consciousness, through its developed intuition is for the first time fully experiencing Spirit and its aspects (immortality and infinite: Compassion, Love, Light, Wisdom, Joy, Peace, Bliss). This experience is of the *Glory* of *Heaven*.

Vishudha   *"Hallowed be thy name"*   *"The Power,"*

Within the orientation of this chakra, the consciousness through its developing intuition is for the first time experiencing large amounts of knowledge and highly developed concepts. This includes the ability to express this information verbally through the throat chakra. The *hallowedness* of the concepts used in understanding, manifesting and naming of Reality is experienced. Reality is Spirit. The profound sacredness of Reality itself is experienced and a deep understanding of *the Power* of God.

Anahata   *"Thy kingdom come"*   *"For thine is the Kingdom,"*

Within the orientation of this chakra, the consciousness through its developing intuition, is for the first time beginning to experience what the *Kingdom* of God is. Through the first three chakra the intuition and consciousness is not developed enough to experience anything beyond what the five senses can perceive. This chakra is the source of our first spiritual insights (our first experiences of universal Love). These phrases are making reference to the developing knowledge and experience of the *Kingdom* of God within the personality orientation of this fourth chakra.

Manipura   *"Thy will be done"*   *"And lead us not into temptation, But deliver us from evil."*

Within the orientation of this chakra and the two lower ones, the consciousness does not have the spiritual maturity to appropriately care about the self and others. The will of the deluded ego, the psychological demons, very often drive the behavior into inappropriateness. This will drive up the karmic debt, dramatically slowing progress and creating stress and suffering. Until the ego surrenders to Spirit there is a possibility of making poor choices. But without much real spiritual experience the possibility is very great. "Thy will be done" is an affirmation of surrender to Spirit.

In the second phrase there could be translation error. God will not lead us into temptation. But this error is a common perception of the spiritually immature personality orientation of the Manipura Chakra. This is the "I am a victim" rationalization. We are always presented with options and we have free will; so the choice is ultimately ours. We choose to allow ourselves to be tempted or not. This phrase is really a request for divine assistance in making appropriate choices.

Taking this a step further, if we allow ourselves to dwell on tempting thoughts, our thoughts will draw into our environmental sphere that which we dwell on. We will attract that which we are imbuing with the energy of our thought. In this way, we are responsible for all our situations and circumstances, good and bad. In order to make progress on the spiritual path it is required that we acknowledge this responsibility and take control of our thoughts and behavior accordingly.

Chakra Correlation of the Phrases within The Lord's Prayer - (continued)

Swadhisthana   *"On Earth as it is in heaven"*.   *"as we forgive those who trespass against us."*

This first phrase is calling our attention to the divine feminine energy symbolized in Eve, the Divine Mother. Also known as the Earth Mother in native American mythologies. The seat of this energy, in humanity, is in this chakra. This energy is just as much a part of heaven as the masculine energy of the Heavenly Father; in this case symbolized as Adam. The seat of this masculine energy in humanity is in the Ajna Chakra. In Christian terminology, the Ajna chakra is the Bridal Chamber. These energies are in humanity *on Earth* just *as they are in Heaven*, in the core of our own beings. In the performance of the Bridal Chamber Sacrament, the energy of Eve is guided from the Swadhisthana Chakra into the Bridal Chamber where these two energies achieve union. A huge amount of energy is released in a spiritual orgasm. The consciousness passes through the Star of the Spiritual Eye and into the Light of Spirit. The result is the birth of Christ (Christ Consciousness).

Within the personality orientation of this chakra, the consciousness first begins to forgive others. Before this orientation we value nothing but ourselves. As we mature into the Swadhisthana orientation we come to realize our dependance on our parents. We realize their value to us and begin to care about their welfare and begin to identify ourselves with them. With this identification we begin to over look perceived minor negligence and as time goes by even major trespasses. Forgiveness is a required component of the Personality Purification Process; *"as we forgive those who trespass against us."*. This second phrase is an affirmation of this requirement to *forgive*.

Mulahara   *" Give us this day our daily bread"*   *" and forgive us our trespasses,"*

Within the orientation of this chakra, the consciousness is obsessed with the physical security of the body. The first phrase is asking for physical sustenance. Symbolically it can also be asking for spiritual sustenance.

Our spiritual ignorance which is the cause of our stress and suffering originate in the personality orientation of this chakra. This is the origin of the trespasses that must be forgiven. Through the use of the Bridal Chamber Sacrament, the purification of consciousness can be facilitated. Grace is involved in this process. Through grace it is possible to receive some assistance with our karmic debt. The second phrase is asking for this assistance. The practice of the more advanced methods of the Bridal Chamber Sacrament begins with this chakra.

"If anyone becomes a child of the Bridal Chamber, he will receive the Light. The one who has received the Light cannot be seen nor can he be held. And no one can torment him, even while he lives in the world. And further, when he goes out of the world, already he has received the Truth."
    The Gnostic Gospel of Philip - verse 127

"They brought forward two evildoers and crucified the Lord between them. But he was silent, as if he had no pain."   The Gnostic Gospel of Peter - verse 10

"These things I have spoken unto you, that in me ye might have peace.
In the world ye shall have tribulation: but be of good cheer; I have overcome the world."
    Jesus - John 16: 33

Salt Water Detoxification
(also called the **Seawater Cleanse**)

Chi kung and Pranayamic techniques will work dramatically better when the body is in optimum health.

The Saltwater Cleanse is a powerful physical cleanse that will clean the entire alimentary canal and even remove accumulating fecal deposits. The average American has five pounds of these deposits in their digestive systems, which is the number one cause of colon cancer in the U.S.. These deposits are a constant source of toxin absorption which causes huge amounts of nutrient and energy depletion and leads to premature ageing and death.

In addition to the alimentary canal cleanse this technique will remove toxins from the blood, enhancing the circulatory system's ability to clean the entire body. Due to effects of osmosis, as the saltwater passes through the small intestines, the electrolytes that the blood needs are absorbed through the villi into the blood. And the toxins in the blood, pass through the villi into the intestines, to be expelled with the excrement. The immune system becomes stronger, reducing all diseases. And with enhanced health comes greater longevity* and the body's ability to hold larger amounts of energy increases*.

A more metaphysical benefit is the results of balancing and matching of the body's electrolyte levels with the oceans of the Earth (seawater). The blood of all the animals on Earth evolved from seawater. Not only do the electrolyte levels of healthy human blood match seawater, but the more perfectly they match, the more energy the body can actually retain. The oceans cover the majority of the planet's surface and hold the vast majority of its life energy, in the form of plankton, its vegetation, animals and fish. The oceans themselves have evolved to hold this energy efficiently. When the human body's electrolyte levels match those of the oceans, it can hold larger amounts of energy too. And with this balance, the human body can even more efficiently access the energy of the Earth.

The Recipe

One quart of lukewarm water (about body temperature)
Mix in two level *teaspoons* of sea salt (no additives, including anti-caking additives)
   This ratio will give you reconstituted seawater.
Drink this down: first thing in the morning, as quickly as possible, before eating or drinking anything else, and stay close to the pot. It will eventually come out like an enema (thirty minutes, beginners usually take a little longer until they get used to it).
It will initially work better if nothing is eaten after 5:00 PM the previous evening.

* Longevity is important to increase the time we have on Earth to take advantage of our spiritual training and to provide service.
* The body's ability to hold larger amounts of energy is important to develop our intuition.
   (see Chakra Influences Page 4-3; Energization of Consciousness)

The value of fasting is evidenced by its use within the spiritual traditions around the world and throughout history. Fasting was prerequisite for many of the Lokota ceremonies especially the Sun Dance, Vision Quest and Sweat Lodge. The Buddha practiced fasting, Jesus fasted forty days and nights in the wilderness and Moses fasted on Mount Sinai. Monks of nearly all sects are advised to fast.

Fasting is used to:
1) detoxify the body: the more toxins in the body the more energy the body must use to maintain itself/ less toxins more energy is available to enhance thought processes and intuition. .
2) shut down digestion; a considerable amount of energy is used for digestion, with nothing to digest a dramatic increase of energy is available to enhance thought processes and intuition.
3) enhance awareness of the separateness of the body, mind and soul.
4) trains self discipline and builds the power of the will.
5) increase mental energy and concentration

It is not healthy to fast more than four days.
Water only, three day fasts are recommended once every three months.
As are one day fasts, once a week.

It is important to stay well hydrated as one fasts. A water only fast will enhance detoxification.
Juice fasts keep sugar levels more stable reducing some side effects that may occur during a fast (low energy levels, headaches, dizziness, body odor, palpitations, sometimes breathing issues).
Fruit can be taken during the fast to remediate side effects. But if palpitations or breathing issues persist the fast should be ended slowly.
The Sea Salt Procedure or an enema is recommended on the first and second day of the fast to enhance detoxification and empty the bowels.
Heart rate slows slightly during fasts. It may be necessary to wear more clothing.
Physical energy levels drop during fasts so strenuous exercise is avoided.

Recommended are the Tai Chi 108, and the Yoga Asana Set; each once a day during the fast. This light exercise aids in detoxification and circulation, in addition to their holistic health benefits.

The additional time gained from not having to eat should be spent meditating and practicing the Crane and Cobra breath.

It is important to break the fast slowly. When fasting the stomach becomes smaller and can not physically hold as much food as one is used to. The first meal should be juicy fruits such as grapes and cherries (do not eat the seeds). Citrus fruits may be too acidic unless the fast was an orange juice fast. Do not over indulge. Nothing more should be eaten until this first meal is fully digested. The next meals should be fruit and vegetable salads for the next day. If the fast is longer than one day, add breads, grains and steamed vegetables to the meals on the third day. And on the fourth day gradually return to your normal diet.

Chi Kung Training Methods — Stretching Introduction

Stretching can also be used as an efficient means of stress management. It will develop flexibility, relaxation skills and act as a warm up preparation for physical activities.

Stretching will assist in physical conditioning of muscles and create suppleness of spine and joints. It will help move lactic acid, that causes muscle stiffness, out of muscles recuperating from strenuous use. It will tone muscles, glands and internal organs. In the east it is believed that the youth of the body is directly related to the flexibility of the spine.

The relaxation after a stretch:
    relieves tension, and counteracts the degenerative effects of stress
    will help to lower levels of glucocorticoids in the body
    assists in the recognition of tension in the body
    enables conscious control of relaxation
    reawakens your awareness and control of your body
    when tension is relieved in the body, the mind is calmed
    moves freshly oxygenated blood into the internal organs relieving tension and stress there
    freshly oxygenated blood will increase mental acuity and clear the thoughts.

Stretching is performed as part of a warm-up preparation for physical activities. It moves freshly oxygenated blood into the muscles to facilitate efficient movement and reduces the potential for strain.

It is recommended that stretching be performed prior to practice of the Crane Breath and daily meditation; especially the <u>spinal center opening sequence</u> and its affirmations. (see next page).

Method of Stretching
    There are three parts of a stretch.

1) move slowly and smoothly into the stretch
2) hold the stretch, gently
   a. at no time stretch into any pain
   b. allow the muscles to relax into the stretch for as long as it is comfortable
   c. a few seconds at first, then longer as it becomes easier with the practice
   d. when holding for any length of time, use the abdominal breath, breath slowly
   e. when practicing with others there should be no competition
3) move slowly and smoothly out of the stretch
   finish relaxed and full of energy

Use a small carpet and/or a blanket.
Wear non-restrictive clothing.
Barefoot is best.

Chi Kung Training Methods   Stretching Routines

Standing

Preparation sequence for physical chi kung training (See Instructional Aids, page D-1 - DVD)

1) standing with half horse stance, torso twist with arm swing, with hand tap at navel and spine
2) standing with half horse stance,
    arms held straight and rotated at shoulder, first forward then reverse
3) neck stretching
    lean the head forward, backward, to the left, to the right, turn it to the left, turn it to the right
4) standing one leg at a time is placed on a stretching bar
5) standing leg swing, 12 reps each leg
6) standing leg extension, bend and left knee, then straighten knee, 5 to 12 reps each leg
7) standing feet together and knees straight, place palms on floor
8) standing feet shoulder width apart, hands on hips, lean back
9) horse stance, hold feet, shift weight into the reverse bow stance,
    with the alternate bending of the knee and straightening of the other

Seated or Laying on Floor

(See Instructional Aids - DVD)

Preparation Sequence for the
    Spinal Center Opening Sequence

1) saint embraces feet
Seated on the floor with the legs straight and together or apart, lean forward and hold feet.
    Or one leg at a time with both hands holding one foot and the other foot placed in and with knee bent.
2) cat
3) cow
4) rocking chair
5) rocking bow

Note: these seated and lying on floor stretches are standard stretching asanas from Hatha Yoga

Spinal Center Opening Sequence:

6) butterfly
7) saint embraces feet/ legs apart
8) prone spinal twist / left and right sides
9) bridge
10) fish
11) seated spinal twist / left and right sides
12) plough
13) shoulder Stand
14) cobra
15) camel

* used to prepare for more efficient energy transportation
*alternate forward and backward bends
*forward spinal bend opens centers,
*backward spinal bend moves energy to higher centers
*performed with mental focus and optionally with mantra and or affirmation

Energization Exercise and Yoga Nidra

This training will develop the ability to achieve total physical relaxation and enhanced energy conservation ability. This state of deep physical relaxation used in conjunction with meditation, can enable the experience of yoga nidra in which it is possible to obtain profound experiences, concepts, ideas, and feelings.

The Benefits

reduces physical tension and stress
raises energy levels
heightens vitality
increases muscle tone
improves concentration

enhances the immune system
physiological processes are strengthened
biologic aging is slowed
regenerative energies are activated
develops proprioceptive sense

General Directions

Laying in the savasana, isolate the tension in each specific part, as the tension is applied.
   Do not tense any other part as you tense the part you are working on.
As the tension is applied, slowly inhale (abdominal breath).
With the inhale of the breath, and an act of will and intention, visualize drawing the energy around you into the tensed body part. When the session is complete, finish in the savasana in deep relaxation and **meditation**.

The Method

Excellent results can be obtained from the first week option alone. It is possible to get a little better results from each subsequent week option. It is easier to learn the sequences if done in this week by week order but not mandatory.

<u>First week</u> at least twice a day. Tense each part (light, medium, and hard) then completely release and relax immediately after each body part is tensed.

<u>Second week</u> at least twice a day, tense each part (light, medium, and hard) and hold. When the whole body is tensed, completely release and relax.

<u>Third week</u> at least twice a day, tense each part (light, medium, and hard) and hold. When the whole body is tensed, completely release and relax each part in reverse order.

<u>Fourth week</u> at least twice a day, tense each part (light, medium, and hard) and hold. When the whole body is tensed, completely release and relax each part in reverse order (hard, medium, light).

Proceed in this order

1) left foot
2) right foot
3) left shin
4) right shin
5) left thigh
6) right thigh
7) left hip
8) right hip
9) lower abdomen
10) upper abdomen
11) left chest
12) right chest
13) left lower back
14) right lower back
15) left upper back
16) right upper back
17) left upper arm and shoulder
18) right upper arm and shoulder
19) left neck
20) right neck
21) back of neck
22) front of neck

Correlation of long term stress symptoms to resulting disease

High levels of chi are required for physical and mental health and the development of spiritual realization. Stress dramatically reduces energy levels resulting in physical and mental deterioration and an inability to perceive Spirit.

Symptoms of the body's response to stress are caused by glucocorticoid hormones secreted into the body by the adrenal glands. Glucocorticoids are steroids; and just like any other steroid or toxin too much of them can poison us. When we are experiencing stress we are literally being poisoned. This will cause symptoms of disease and aging. It is important that we learn to control this response to stress.

Stress Symptom	Resulting Disease
mobilized energy, diabetes, bruxism	fatigue, muscle destruction,
Increased cardiovascular activity	hypertension, enlarged heart
suppressed digestion	ulceration, colitis, irritable bowel syndrome
suppressed reproduction	impotence, loss of libido, interruption of menstruation
suppression of immune response	increased risk of disease: colds, flu, cancer, etc.
sharpening of thought and perception	neuron damage or death

The Symptoms Produced by Steroid Poisoning

are also the symptoms produced by too much stress and aging

muscle wasting	thinning skin	hypertension
diabetes	redistribution of body fat	impaired mental function
fatigue	fragility of blood vessels	suppression of immune function
osteoporosis	fluid retention	

Breath: Introductory Information

It is the perceptions of the mind that cause stress. This can easily be shown by the fact that the same situation or circumstance will elicit the stress response in one person and not in another. If we can control the mind we can also control the levels of stress we experience. Control of the breath will assist in the control of the mind.

The breath and the mind are inseparable. The condition of one will influence the condition of the other. Shallow short breathing, that can occur spontaneously when we are anxious, excites and agitates the mind making one upset, dizzy and or fatigued. This will initiate the body's stress responses.

Slow deep breathing will calm the mind.

An on the spot anxiety reducing technique is to take a few slow deep breaths. As you breath in, fill the bottom of the lungs first, then the chest and then raise the shoulders. This will leave you calmer and in more control.

Control of the breath is used in the practice of the San Zan form to substantially enhance the energization and energy balancing effects of the exercise.

Control of the breath will assist in:
- control of anxiety produced by stress
- slowing of the aging process
- raising levels of vitality
- training the conscious transportation of chi
- reaching the advanced levels of spiritual awareness

The Abdominal Breathing Technique

This is the first breathing technique that we will use for practice of Chi Kung or Pranayama. It is sometimes called the Buddhist breath or postnatal breathing. You will need to train yourself to breath into your stomach. The shoulders stay down, the chest does not move. The lower abdomen expands with the inhale and contracts with the exhale.

The abdominal breath more efficiently oxidizes the blood allowing more air to come in. The average untrained breath will bring in about one pint of air. An average trained abdominal breath can be three pints, actually allowing the breathing rate to slow.

In the east it is believed that efficient breathing will extend the life time.

The Four Part Abdominal Breath

The four part abdominal breathing technique is used in San Zan and in some meditation techniques. The four parts of the breath are:
1) The inhale
2) The hold of the breath with the abdomen 90% full
3) The exhale
4) The hold of the breath with the abdomen 90% empty

Practice usually begins seated, spine straight, chin level, body relaxed as possible, eyes closed and the gaze gently raised to the spot between the eyebrows. This exercise has a powerful calming effect and for this reason it is sometimes used to begin meditation practice.

Practice of the four part breath begins with 3 counts for each breath part.

Practice everyday, increasing to 6 counts; then longer as comfort allows.

Chi Kung Training Methods   The Crane Breath

The Crane Breath

    The Crane Breath is the first chi/prana accumulation technique presented in Tamo's Muscle and Tendon Changing Methods. This is an abdominal breath that uses a visualization to assist in the transportation and accumulation of chi/prana. The visualization is used in combination with mental concentration and an act of will to make the transportation of energy to occur. The practice of this technique will enhance the immune system and increase vitality levels, mental acuity and intuition. The beginner is encouraged to practice this with at least eighteen breaths prior to meditating, daily.

1) Seated in the Zen Meditation Posture (knees and insteps on floor and seated on the heals) or cross legged or any comfortable seated position.
Place the hands in the lap. Hold the spine straight but not strained,
jaw level, shoulders back, chest box forward. With the back straight, allow the body to relax. Gently place the tip of the tongue on the roof of the mouth.

2) With the eyes closed, raise the gaze to the spot between the eye brows and without any strain gently hold the gaze toward this spot as this exercise is performed. (note 1)

3) Breath abdominally, using only the diaphragm. The shoulders stay down and the chest should not move at all. The stomach should expand with the inhale and contract with the exhale. Be careful not to breath too much air in or too much air out; make this breath comfortable and slow.

4) This energization exercise begins by visualizing the inhaling of the energy in the air around the body, through the mouth with the breath. Using mental focus and an act of will, visualize the energy entering the mouth with the breath, absorbing into the back of the tongue and traveling down the front centerline of the body (note 2) into the navel center (note 3).
The navel center is located in the abdomen, two or three inches behind the navel.

5) As the air is exhaled, visualize the energy that was inhaled with the breath, being accumulated and stored in the navel center.

(Note 1) This spot is called the Upper Tan Tien. Looking into it with the eyes closed is called the Frontal Gaze. This will assist in the focus of the Yi (intention, the will, the Wisdom Mind), which is required for efficient chi/prana transportation.
(Note 2) This is the acupuncture meridian, the Conception Vessel. This vessel runs from the tip of the tongue, down the front centerline of the torso, to the Huiyin Cavity at the base of the torso. It also connects to the Lower Tan Tien as it passes the navel.
(Note 3) The navel center is the Lower Tan Tien. This Tan Tien acts as a storage battery for energy in the human body. The Tan Tien will distribute energy to the body for health and vitality via the Conception Vessel and the Governing Vessel. The Governing Vessel runs from the roof of the mouth up the centerline of the face, over the crest of the head and down the centerline of the back where it connects to the Conception Vessel; again at the Huiyin Cavity at the base of the torso.

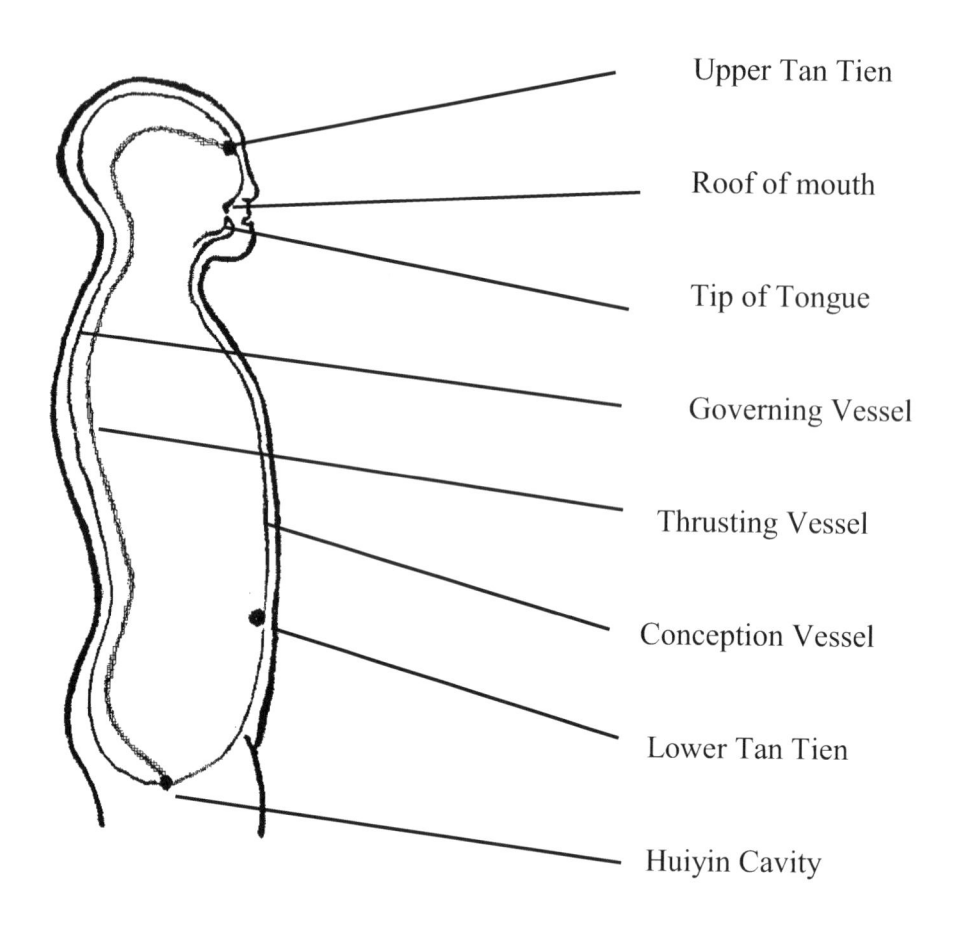

- Upper Tan Tien
- Roof of mouth
- Tip of Tongue
- Governing Vessel
- Thrusting Vessel
- Conception Vessel
- Lower Tan Tien
- Huiyin Cavity

Components Used In Consciousness Energization

The Upper Tan Tien is the Ajna Chakra of Yogic Mysticism. Its center is associated with the pituitary gland. The Upper Tan Tien is the organ of intuition in humanity. Gently raising the gaze toward this spot between the eye brows and holding the mental attention here will energize this astral organ and heighten the intuitional ability. The gaze into it is called the Frontal Gaze. The Upper Tan Tien is also the command center for the transportation of Chi. This gaze will assist in the focus of the Yi (intention, the will, the Wisdom Mind), which is required for efficient chi transportation during meditation and in the practice of the Crane Breath and the Cobra Breath.

The Lower Tan Tien is known as the Manapura Chakra in Yogic Mysticism and the Hara in Japanese. It is located 2 or 3 inches behind the naval and connects to the Conception Vessel in front and the Thrusting Vessel in the back.

The Thrusting Vessel runs from the Upper Tan Tien between the two hemispheres of the brain, through the medulla, down the center of the spinal cord and terminates with the Conception and Governing Vessels at the Huiyin Cavity. This is the path used for Cobra Breath training.

Chi Kung Training Methods
The Mystical Meaning of the Mudra and Movements of *San Zan*

San Zan is a pranayama/chi kung exercise taught within the Shaolin Tradition. Exercises like this are called forms (hsing in Chinese, kata in Japanese and nata in Sanskrit). They are a sequence of movements and postures which include mudra and/or martial technique. These pranayama/chi kung methods have been practiced within the yogic tradition of India well into prehistoric times. Some evidence suggests 4000 B.C.. Bodhidharma, is known as: the 28th patriarch of Buddhism, the 1st patriarch of Chan sect of Buddhism (Zen in Japan), and the founder of the Shaolin Tradition. Chan is the Chinese shorten form of the word chan'na which means meditation. Chan'na is the mispronunciation of the Sanskrit word dhyana (meditation). Bodhidharma was responsible for reintroducing meditation into Buddhism after it had fallen out of use for centuries. He introduced meditation and three forms to the monks at the Shaolin Temple in China in 525 A.D.. These forms are San Zan (Tri Can in Sanskrit), Sei San Chuan and San Sei Chuan. These three forms come from the Vajramukti Yoga system which is a Hindu sect of yogic mysticism. They are very ancient and predate Bodhidharma by many centuries.

San Zan uses mudra, affirmations, movement, physical tension and breath control for the purpose of developing spiritual awareness. It accomplishes this by:
1) developing physical strength for the stamina required for long periods of meditation. Secondary physical benefits are an extraordinary immune system and extended longevity.
2) raising energy levels: a) to develop the intuition (intuition is required to obtain results from meditation), b) enhances mental abilities to comprehend concepts, techniques and methods used to develop spiritual awareness, c) to mentally stay on task and focused for long periods of time (required for meditation), d) develops the power of the will required to achieve the goal.
3) teaching spiritual concepts through mudra that are vital for developing spiritual awareness.
4) building and sustaining motivational levels so that the results of the training can be realized.
5) Samasthana training. Samasthana is self examination/personality purification used to expose the sthana to the self for the removal of the orientation to duality. The sthana is the personality; its belief system (its orientation to duality, the worldly paradigm, its limitations, delusions and illusions) and the resulting thought and behavior patterns.

Bodhidharma called San Zan the Eighteen Hands of Avatars. His thought was that the practice of this form would turn the lohan into avatars. But after he left the temple the monks thought that since only lohans practiced the form it should be called the Eighteen Hands of the Lohan. This name was used for some centuries. In the form there are eighteen formal energization breaths that are coordinated with mudra, affirmations and movements of the hands. The monks at the Fukien Shaolin Temple started to call the form San Zan; probably because it was easier to say. San Zan is Chinese for Three Battles. Three Battles metaphorically has two meanings. The first refers to the process of personality purification used to remove the three klesa (self-centeredness, spiritual ignorance, and fear) from the personality. The second meaning is addressing the process of experiencing the union of the self, duality, and Spirit. This experience is part of the experience of enlightenment. It was the Okinawans that took the mudra out of the form and called it Sanchin. Sanchin is the Okinawan mispronunciation of San Zan, but it has the same meaning. The Okinawans would only show and explain the consciousness energization methods, mudra and meanings of the form to mystically prepared initiates.

4 - 24 Chi Kung Training Methods
The Mystical Meaning of the Mudra and Movements of San Zan (continued)

The first movement of San Zan starts with the Namaste Mudra and a bow. This mudra is a declaration of Truth that the Infinite Eternal Life of Love and Compassion exits within the self, all others, all of Creation and Spirit. The bow is a show of supreme respect for Spirit.

The second set of movements are: the double exhale, the assumption of the vajra bu (the lightning bolt stance), the double presentation of the Bhumisparsha Mudra and the double presentation of Abaya Mudra with the slow inhale using the ujaiya breath. The movements end with the "E exhale" of the Cobra Breath and the return to the double Bhumisparsha Mudra.

The vajra bu is obtained simultaneously with the double exhale. In the vajra bu stance, the jagged lines in the placement of the body's appendages represent exploding bolts of lightning. The vajra bu is called the hour glass stance by those that do not understand the lightning bolt metaphor. Probably because the position of the forearms, elbows, knees and thighs make it look a little like an hour glass. But the lightning bolt represents the super high energy levels the practice of San Zan will instill in the being of the practitioner. When in the proximity of a cracking lightning bolt the light emitted is blinding, brighter than the Sun. This is the brilliance of the Light of Spirit experienced when the intuitional awareness rises through the Sound of Creation (Omm) and into the direct experience of Pure Spirit. And with this experience explodes the awareness of Unity and all the aspects of Spirit. This is the experience of enlightenment. It is through the intuition that we obtain this experience. The intuition requires super high levels of energy to enable the apprehension of this experience. Intuitional ability is directly proportional to energy levels. It is the practice of San Zan that presents the potential to acquire these levels of energy and this experience.

The double exhale is a cleansing breath used to prepare the body for spiritual cleansing and energization, in the performance of San Zan. It also empties the lungs for the first energizing breath. The double presentation of the Bhumisparsha Mudra, the gesture of "touching the Earth", is the gesture that the Buddha performed when he made the Divine Mother aware of his initial experience of God Realization while meditating under the banyan tree. It has come to indicate that what is being said is Truth and is unchangeable as Truth. This is similar to what one of the uses of the word Omm has come to mean in Buddhism and Hinduism and what Amen has come to mean in Christianity. The double presentation of the Abaya Mudra begins and ends with the Bhumisparsha Mudra indicating the Truth that the Abaya Mudra represents.

The Abaya Mudra is a request for divine assistance in the incorporation of Divine Peace, and Fearlessness (and the aspects of Spirit) into ones personality. It is also a statement of Truth, "I am an immortal spiritual being of Peace and Fearlessness". This concept of fearlessness is aimed at the courage required to face and defeat the klesic demons of self centeredness, ignorance (recognizing the delusion of duality), and fear in the process of personality purification. This victory is prerequisite for complete spiritual realization. With the defeat of the inner demons, one becomes a being on Infinite Peace. Peace is usually the first aspect of Spirit experienced by the aspiring mystic. As Divine Peace is experienced it will blossom into an experience of all the aspects of Spirit and in this case Peace represents them all. This mudra becomes a sign of non-aggression, protection, blessing, reassurance and compassion for all others.

Chi Kung Training Methods
The Mystical Meaning of the Mudra and Movements of San Zan (continued)

The personality must be purified to completely experience Spirit. The amount of spiritual realization one attains is directly proportional to how well the aspects of Spirit are integrated into the personality. The integration of Spirit into the personality is the function of meditation. Some aspects of Spirit include: Divine Love, Light, Compassion, Truth, Wisdom, Joy, Peace, Unity, Bliss, Omm.

The ujaiya inhale is incorporated into the slow controlled Crane Breath as in the performance of the Abaya Mudra. This inhale is used to enhance the energization effects of the Crane Breath. The "E exhale" is used to enhance the personality purification effects of the Cobra Breath. The energizing breath used is either the Crane Breath or the Cobra Breath, depending on what level of training the practitioner is at.

As we face the east we are exposing ourselves to the pranic/chi currents blowing across the face of the Earth from that direction. Prana/chi is the energy of Spirit manifesting in Creation. It permeates outer space, our atmosphere, all of Creation. The blowing of this energy occurs due to the rotation of the surface of the Earth into the east. The prana/chi is blowing into our faces as we face east. Facing east, we expose our energy collecting orifices (mouth, nose, eyes, ears) and in this case additionally the small chakra, the Labor Palace, located in the center of the palms of the hands. This is why we face the east when we meditate and perform forms. As we perform the Abaya Mudra, with the palms of the hands facing the east, we can open the Labor Palace and suck additional energy into our being, visualizing this with the inhale of the breath.

The third set of movements are the right arcing step into a right foot forward vajra bu and the lightning fast double presentation of the Bhumisparsha Mudra and the Buddha Shramana Mudra. As explained earlier, the Bhumisparsha Mudra is used to enhance the credibility of the meaning of an associated mudra, in this case the Buddha Shramana. The Buddha Shramana mudra represents a commitment to not participate in the competition for resources, security, power, authority or survival that is predominate in the cultures and social norms of the world (the worldly paradigm). This mudra is the affirmation of the renunciant, "I am an immortal spiritual being, while I live in this world, I will not be part of it". This mudra also represents the realization of existing in a state beyond the stress and suffering of the world. This realization comes with the experience of not being part of this world. To become fully aware of not being part of the world requires an experience of enlightenment.

The fourth set of movements are: the first set of five forward arcing steps, coordinating a formal energizing breath with each step, and movements of the arms performing the Bhumisparsha Mudra, Buddha Shramana Mudra and the Varada Mudra. The first five steps include a set of affirmations dedicated to the incorporation of the Five Perfections into the personality of the practitioner. One of these affirmations is recited with each step. Between each step a formal energizing breath is taken, coordinating the breath with arm movements used to perform each mudra. The movement of the arms also trace the movement of the accumulating energy within the torso and head. This assists the efficient accumulation and transportation of energy within the practitioners astral being. When these methods are used with the 5 Perfections Affirmations, they will assist in the Purification of Consciousness; training personality purification and energization of consciousness.

Chi Kung Training Methods
The Mystical Meaning of the Mudra and Movements of San Zan (continued)

The Bhumisparsha Mudra and the Buddha Shramana Mudra are intrinsic to these sets of movements because San Zan is an exercise of living as "not part of the world". The San Zan form is an exercise that will actually move the practitioner out of the worldly paradigm, when practiced by a sincere, disciplined, aspiring mystic. These sets of movements and affirmations were intentionally designed to make this experience possible.

The Varada Mudra represents the acquisition of the supreme accomplishment; the complete integration of the Five Perfections into the conscious awareness (the supreme accomplishment results in illumination). Each of the five fingers represents one of the Five Perfections. The Five Perfections is an ancient template used in the Process of Personality Purification for the development of spiritual awareness. This mudra is also a request for divine assistance in the acquisition of the supreme accomplishment. The affirmation of this mudra is "I am an immortal spiritual being, transformed by the Five Perfections, I am devoted to the salvation of humanity."

The Five Perfections

1) Perfect Compassion develops Perfect Charity
2) Perfect Love develops Perfect Morality
3) Perfect Determination develops Perfect Patience
4) Perfect Discipline develops Perfect Effort
5) Given the first four perfections;
   Perfect Concentration/Meditation results in Illumination

The fifth set of movements are: a step across 180° turn to the left, with the performance of the Buddha Shramana Mudra, Bhumisparsha Mudra and the Varada Mudra, the return to the Vadra Bu stance, and a repeat of the forth set of movements coordinated with the five formal energization breaths. This second set of five steps include a set of affirmations dedicated to the incorporation of the Five Perfections into the *mental* being of the practitioner. Each step includes an affirmation and the same arm movements, mudra and energization breath; with the same use and meanings.

The sixth set of movements are a repeat of the fifth set of movements without the steps. This set includes: the step across, 180° turn to the left which places the performer in the exact same place, same stance and facing east, that were used at the beginning of the form. This is the spot where San Zan will end. Most Shaolin forms begin and end at the same spot. This third set of five formal energization breaths include a set of affirmations dedicated to the incorporation of the Five Perfections into the *spiritual* being of the practitioner. The formal energization breaths of the sixth set includes the new set of affirmations and the same arm movements and mudra of the fifth set.

Chi Kung Training Methods
The Mystical Meaning of the Mudra and Movements of San Zan (continued)

The seventh set of movements are performed with the same stance, and only three formal energization breaths. The same mudra are used but instead of the arm movements occurring one at a time, the arm movements are identical and simultaneous. The mudra and movements have the same use and meanings as those of the fourth, fifth and sixth movement sets. Again the affirmations are coordinated with the breaths but they are directed toward the defeat of the klesa.

The klesa are three psychological demons that stand in the way of our spiritual development. These three klesa are: self centeredness, spiritual ignorance and fear. The klesa are a manifestation of the worldly paradigm (maya, in Sanskrit,).

The five formal energization breaths and the arm and hand movements of the fourth, fifth and sixth set of movements, and the three from the seventh, total eighteen. These are the formal eighteen hand movements mentioned in Bodhidharma's original name for the form "The Eighteen Hands of the Avatars". Eighteen is a factor of 108 (6 x18 = 108). Monks are expected to do 108 daily repetitions of the Cobra personality purification / consciousness energization Breath, to make adequate progress with their meditation. One round of eighteen with each of six meditation sittings each day. An alternate daily meditation schedule is three meditation sittings with two rounds of eighteen breaths, included with longer actual meditation time. Among the many other purposes of the form, Bodhidarma used it to teach the newly initiated monks their first round of the Cobra Breath. Meditation and San Zan, then and now, are required for monastic initiation into the Shaolin Sanga.

The eighth set of movements is the San Sao Mudra with a step back with the right leg. The San Sao Mudra is actually the simultaneous performance of three mudra. The Abaya Mudra and Varada Mudra are rotated into a circle. The rotating circle is the third mudra, the Dharma Chakra Mudra. In the performance of the circle, the mudra of each hand reverses into the opposite mudra, then both are pushed out from the centerline of the torso about twelve inches.

The Dharma Chakra Mudra is Sanskrit and translates as, the turning of the cosmic wheel. The turning of the cosmic wheel refers to the balancing of karma that results in constructive experience. This mudra is a request for divine assistance in the process of personality purification and dissolution of the karmic debt. It will bring into your life situations and circumstances that will expose the limitations within your personality that must be eliminated. The exposure enables each limitation to be identified for removal. Conscious effort and an act of will are required for the removal of each limitation from thought and behavior. Eventually, the delusions of ignorance are transformed by the integration of wisdom within the imagined self, into the Wisdom of the Great Self. The affirmation of the San Sao Mudra is "In Perfect Peace I walk the path of the Five Perfections". The capitalization of Perfect and Peace make this a reference to Spirit since Perfect Peace is an aspect of Spirit. The result of walking the path of the Five Perfections is the supreme accomplishment, union with Spirit.

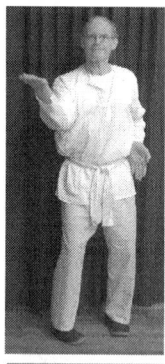

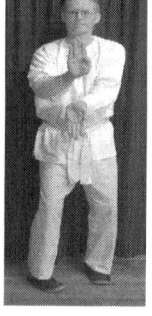

Chi Kung Training Methods
The Mystical Meaning of the Mudra and Movements of San Zan (continued)

The ninth set of movements are: the Dharma-Megha Mudra, the Bhujang Mudra, the double presentation of the Bhumisparsha Mudra and the Abaya Mudra, the Namaste Mudra, and the Bow.

The double presentation of the Bhumisparsha Mudra and the Abaya Mudra, the Namaste Mudra, and the Bow are in the reverse order of the opening movements. These mudra have the same meaning as their use in the opening of the form, but here they are used for the closing.

In the Dharma-Megha Mudra the right arm draws a large ellipse in front of and pretty much outlining the torso. This symbolizes the dissolution of the karmic debt and worldly attachment (which includes the attachment to and awareness, of the self) into the ether. The karmic debt and attachment are the cause of bondage and limitation. With this removal the soul spreads its wings of Wisdom as it is released from maya and rises into the radiant brilliance of Spirit and awareness of all its aspects. The release from maya is also the total release from all stress and suffering and the realization of the supreme accomplishment. The Dharma-Megha Mudra closes with the Bhujang Mudra.

Bhujang is Chinese for the cobra snake. The cobra snake represents the spinal cord, medulla, and the brain because of the similarity in appearance. These are the principal organs used in the Shaolin methods of consciousness energization (ex. San Zan, Cobra Breath, meditation). The Bhujang Mudra represents the methods of the Shaolin Tradition. The energization of the consciousness is required to enhance the intuitional ability to the level required to obtain a direct experience of Spirit (the supreme accomplishment). The affirmation of this mudra is "I am a Shaolin Bodhisattva Monk, using the methods of the Shaolin Tradition to obtain complete God Realization". The Dharma-Megha Mudra represents the goal of the aspiring mystic and the Bhujang Mudra represents the method.

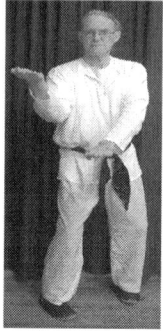

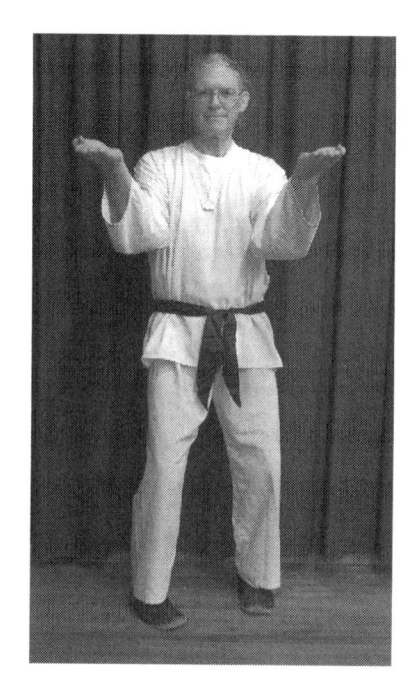

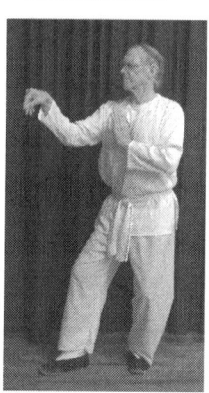

Stance - Posture   (these positions energize the posture)

- The spine is held straight
    (the straight spine allows energy in the body to move more efficiently)
- Chin and gaze level
- The feet are positioned:
    shoulder width apart, heal to toe
    back foot points straight ahead
    front foot and front knee point 45 degrees inward
    the toes are spread
    the feet grab the floor and pull inward   (Done correctly, this will tilt the hips
        forward, further straightening the back, particularly the lower back)
- Both knees are held visibly bent, with the knees over the toes
- The open hands are held shoulder height and just outside the shoulders
- Elbows are held inside the shoulders. Forearms and elbows point at the naval.
    (enhances the internalness of this exercise)
- The anal sphincter muscles are tensed and raised
- Tension is held throughout the body, about 60%
    (attracts energy into the limbs and body, and stimulates overall body strength)

Breath

- Abdominal breath
    (this will assist the lower tan-tien in its function as a storage center for energy,
        opening this chakra for efficient energy transportation)
- Four part (each part of the breath cycle should last the same amount of time)
    1) inhale
    2) hold breath with lower abdomen 90% full
    3) exhale
    4) hold breath with lower abdomen 90% empty
- Breath is coordinated with the arm movements
    (inhale as the arms are brought in; exhale as the arms are pushed out)

Stepping

- Forward and backward stepping are performed with an inward arching step
    (enhances internalness of this exercise)
- The step is performed quickly, keeping the foot as close to the floor as possible
    (do not rise as the step is taken)
- With each step the foot placement, stance, posture and root is regained instantly
    (as the foot is placed)

The Affirmations of San Zan - The Path of the Five Perfections

1) I inhale and imbue this physical being with the energy of perfect Compassion
and with this energy I develop perfect Charity
2) I inhale and imbue this physical being with the energy of perfect Love
and with this energy I develop perfect Morality
3) I inhale and imbue this physical being with the energy of perfect Determination
and with this energy I develop perfect Patience.
4) I inhale and imbue this physical being with the energy of perfect Discipline
and with this energy I develop perfect Effort
5) I inhale and imbue this physical being with the energy of perfect Concentration
and with this energy I discover Zen
6) I inhale and imbue this mental being with the energy of perfect Compassion
and with this energy I develop perfect Charity
7) I inhale and imbue this mental being with the energy of perfect Love
and with this energy I develop perfect Morality
8) I inhale and imbue this mental being with the energy of perfect Determination
and with this energy I develop perfect Patience.
9) I inhale and imbue this mental being with the energy of perfect Discipline
and with this energy I develop perfect Effort
10) I inhale and imbue this mental being with the energy of perfect Concentration
and with this energy I discover Zen
11) I inhale and imbue this spiritual being with the energy of perfect Compassion
and with this energy I develop perfect Charity
12) I inhale and imbue this spiritual being with the energy of perfect Love
and with this energy I develop perfect Morality
13) I inhale and imbue this spiritual being with the energy of perfect Determination
and with this energy I develop perfect Patience.
14) I inhale and imbue this spiritual being with the energy of perfect Discipline
and with this energy I develop perfect Effort
15) I inhale and imbue this spiritual being with the energy of perfect Concentration
and with this energy I discover Zen
16) I inhale and imbue the totality of this being with Supreme Energy
and with this energy I defeat the klesic demon of self-centeredness (narcissism)
17) I inhale and imbue the totality of this being with Supreme Energy
and with this energy I defeat the klesic demon of ignorance
18) I inhale and imbue the totality of this being with Supreme Energy
and with this energy I defeat the klesic demon of fear

In Perfect Peace I walk the Path of the Five Perfections.

With the defeat of the klesas I experience: Spiritual Unity, Love, Light, Compassion, Truth, Wisdom, Joy, and Peace.

Sei San Chuan Diagram and Performance Information

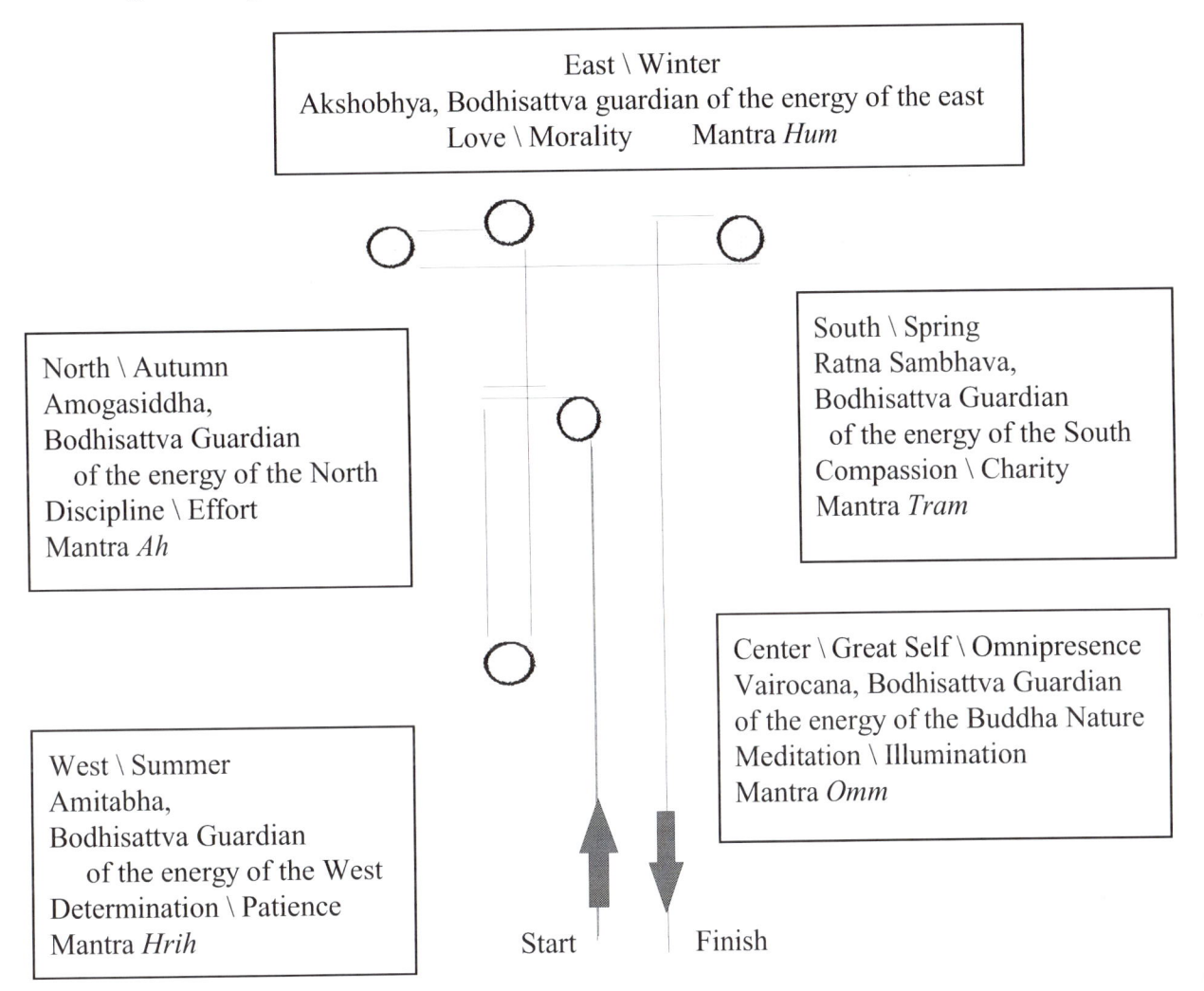

```
                    East \ Winter
    Akshobhya, Bodhisattva guardian of the energy of the east
                Love \ Morality    Mantra Hum
```

North \ Autumn
Amogasiddha,
Bodhisattva Guardian
   of the energy of the North
Discipline \ Effort
Mantra *Ah*

South \ Spring
Ratna Sambhava,
Bodhisattva Guardian
   of the energy of the South
Compassion \ Charity
Mantra *Tram*

Center \ Great Self \ Omnipresence
Vairocana, Bodhisattva Guardian
of the energy of the Buddha Nature
Meditation \ Illumination
Mantra *Omm*

West \ Summer
Amitabha,
Bodhisattva Guardian
   of the energy of the West
Determination \ Patience
Mantra *Hrih*

Start   Finish

The performance of this form is a commitment to the use of the Five Perfections.

The form starts and finishes facing the East. The circles represent the place within the form, that the leap and step-into-merge with the energy of its represented direction, are performed. The leaps are performed with the: visualization of the merge, the mudra set (Abaya and Bhumisparsha), the mantra and usually with an inhale to accumulate the energy and influence of the direction. The Labor Place (the small chakra in the center of the palms of the hands) is used for energy accumulation in conjunction with the Abaya Mudra.

The form starts with the San Zan beginning mudra and breath. Then three formal San Zan forward steps, with San Zan breaths, using the Vajra-bu. The affirmations of the mudra and breath are directed at energizing and illuminating each of the bodies of the performer: the physical body, mental body and astral body. Then a set of three Bumisparsha Mudra "touching the earth" and an associated additional mudra set, are again, directed toward each body.

The form ends with three formal backward stepping San Sao Breaths. Again, the affirmations of the mudra and one breath are directed at energizing and illuminating each of the bodies of the performer: the physical body, mental body and astral body.

4-32 Chi Kung Training Methods   San Sei Chuan Diagram and Performance Information

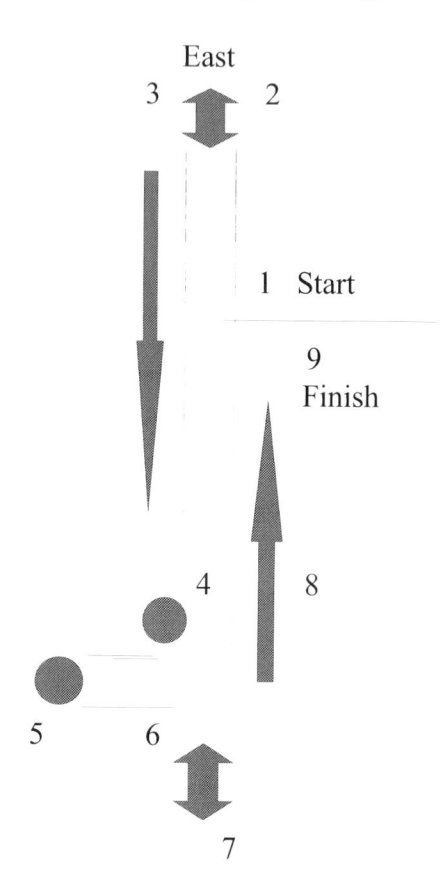

East

3 2

1 Start

9 Finish

4 8

5 6

7

The main objective of this form is spiritual: consciousness energization, personality purification and illumination.
a) Purpose of energization is meditation enhancement
b) This form trains wu-hsin for meditation enhancement
c) There are Mudra with every step and position
d) Multiple San Zan and San Sao and
     energization breath with mudra

A secondary objective of the form is
     the development martial ability.
a) technique and combination performance
b) mobility training
c) defense and counter strategies

The performance of this form is a personal commitment to the complete spiritual evolution of one's own consciousness.

The form starts and finishes facing the East.
The lines represent the path of movement.
The double arrows are 180° turns.
The single arrows are the direction of movement.
The circles represent the places within the form that the leap, step-into and collection of energy are performed.
The leaps are performed with the visualization of the energy collection and
     the mudra set (Abaya and Bhumisparsha).
The Labor Place (the small chakra in the center of the palms of the hands) is used for energy collection in conjunction with the leap and the performance of the Abaya and Bhumisparsha Mudra.

Chi Kung Training Methods
San Sei Chuan Diagram and Performance Information (continued)

The Movement Sequence Each number corresponds to its placement in the diagram.

1) The form starts with three formal forward stepping San Zan breaths with mudra, using the Vajra-bu. The affirmations of the mudra and one breath are directed at energizing each of the bodies of the performer: the physical body, mental body and astral body.

2) Then: an energy accumulation hand rotation technique, double stab, pull and double stomp.
   These first two items, on this list, symbolize the preparation and commitment required to begin walking this spiritual path. The experience of spiritual illumination is unbearable to one who is not prepared. An unprepared human body can experience huge amounts of physical and mental pain and agony for years as the required amounts of energy are experienced. It is the Cobra Breath that is used to accomplish this required preparation.

3) A 180° turn into the West and five Wan-bu steps; with the Nataraja mudra.
   This symbolizes the commitment and the process required to use the Five Perfections as a templet for the spiritual evolution of one's consciousness.

4) A leap into North in ma-bu; with energy collection and three crane punches.
   Items 4, 5, and 6 symbolize the defeat of the three klesa. Self-centeredness is the first. Its defeat is required before the second klesa can be efficiently confronted.

5) A Stomp and leap into the South in ma-bu; with energy collection and two crane punches,
   This symbolizes the attach and defeat of the second klesa, ignorance. Which is the recognition that the worldly paradigm is delusion and is the cause of virtually all stress and suffering. This must be accomplished before the third klesa can be efficiently defeated.

6) A Stomp and leap into the West, recovering a wan-bu facing West; delivering a rising elbow strike, back knuckle strike, double deflection blocks and back knuckle strike combination.
   This combination symbolizes the annihilation of the klesa of fear. This process must be started before one can move through the forth and fifth dimensional orientations.

7) A 180° turn to the East and two forward Wan-bu steps; with the mudra set Buddha-Shramana/Bhumisparsha.
   These steps symbolize the movement of the consciousness thru the 4th and 5th dimensions.

8) Three formal forward stepping San Sao breaths with mudra and Vajra-bu.
   Again, the San Sao affirmations, mudra and one breath are directed at energizing and purifying each of the bodies of the performer: the physical body, mental body and astral body. This energization and purification must be accomplished before step nine can be experienced.

9) The form closes with the Dharma Megha Mudra. This mudra is a commitment to and symbolizes the accomplishment of, complete spiritual illumination.

Chi Kung Training Methods
The Mystical Meaning of the Mudra and Movements of Pai He Chuan

The Movement and Mudra of Pai He Chuan

This form has all the characteristics of the northern Shaolin forms. This indicates that it was most probably created at the original Shaolin Temple in Honan, in northeast China. Its creation certainly occurred before the Shaolin Priest Chang San Feng created the Tai Chi 108, 1200 A.D., since most of its movements and mudra were incorporated into the 108. It was most probably created around 800 A.D.. Originally it was called Pai He Chuan (The form of the Ancient Wisdom of the White Crane). Obviously it was called this because of all the Crane related movement and strategies within it, but also because it was physical and mental training intended to prepare the monks for the spiritual training. Physical and mental training intended to prepare the monks for spiritual training was called White Crane training.

Possibly centuries later, the name was shortened to Chinto. This was the name used at the Shaolin Temple at Fukien, in southeast China. The Okinawans learned this form as Chinto, when they were taught it at the Fukien Temple during the 16th and 17th centuries. Chinto means "To Face the East". This is auspicious because the Shaolin forms were intended to be forms of moving meditation. It is important to face the East, during meditation, to take advantage of the chi/prana energy moving across the surface of our planet as it turns into the East. The Earth spins at about 1000 miles an hour at the equator. All of Creation, our universe and all the space between the celestial bodies are made of and permeated by chi/prana. High energy levels are required to meditate efficiently. It is possible to absorb this chi/prana energy as it blows into the orifices on our faces and through our skin as it comes at us from the East. All the Shaolin forms and meditation begin and end facing the East.

The practice of Chinto will develop the intense mental focus required to meditate efficiently. This is especially noticeable in the performance of the one leg crane stances and the combinations of movements associated with them. The coordination required for the flying front kick, the precision of movement and posture changes, speed, and alternating tension and relaxation also requires the development of this mental focus.

Once the meaning of the mudra are understood, the practice of this form will enhance: spiritual insight, energy levels, an appreciation for the spiritual training, the motivation for continued training.

When the Shaolin Monks had completed their training at the temple, they were expected to travel through China mediating disagreements, generally helping to maintain the Peace and making the spiritual teachings available to those who could use them. The ultimate goal of the Shaolin Tradition was not just to train a compassionate police force and judicial system, it was to develop a large body of fully enlightened beings that could efficiently assist in the spiritual evolution of humanity: a huge organization of Bodhisattvas. For over a thousand years Chinto has been an integral part of the training used to achieve this goal.

Chi Kung Training Methods
The Mystical Meaning of the Mudra and Movements of Pai He Chuan (continued)

Movement number: Each number represents a set of movements performed in this order within the form. When the form is practiced in a group, the movements described within each number are performed with a beat of a drum.

1. Facing east with the gaze leveled there,
the right foot steps back to the wan-bu (bow stance),
delivering an overhead cross-arm block with the fists (Double Dhrithi Mudra)
that then open into the Double Abaya Mudra.

    The Dhrithi Mudra is used to declare a total commitment to one or more mudra associated with it. This Double Dhrithi Mudra represents the total commitment to the mudra that follows. The Abaya Mudra represents Peace and Fearlessness. It is a statement of good intentions. The left and right hand of the double Abaya Mudra, also represent the Yin and Yang Creative energies of the Tiger and Dragon. The Tiger represents the Yin Energy of the feminine divine creative energy, the Divine Mother and Vishnu. The Dragon represents the Yang Energy of the masculine divine creative energy, the Heavenly Father and Shiva. Presented together they represent the: Shaolin Tradition, Tao, Brahma and Unity with the Great Spirit.

2. Continue with the gaze facing east.
The weight shifts backward into the bao-bu (cat stance).
Performed in this order is the: San Sao Mudra to the Heavens, left hammer fist, right reverse crane punch.

    The San Sao Mudra originally came from the San Zan form. In the Tai Chi 108 it became the *Ward Off* movement.

    The San Sao Mudra is a request for divine assistance in the process of personality purification, the dissolution of the karmic debt and the process of illumination.

    The delivery of the left and right fists is an emphatic double presentation of the Dhrithi Mudra of the Closed Fist. The Dhrithi Mudra expresses the meaning of the 3rd and 4th perfections of the Five Perfections of the Shaolin Tradition. The third perfection is Perfect Determination and Patience and the fourth is Perfect Discipline and Effort. The performance of the Dhrithi Mudra here represents the total commitment to the meaning of the San Sao Mudra and the previous mudra presentation of the Double Abaya Mudra and its meaning.

3. The head turns left as the gaze is leveled to the west.
Pivot 180 degrees to the left, on the left foot, stepping with the right, into ma-bu (horse stance, this stance squares off facing south but the head and gaze is leveled west).
Deliver a low block to the west with the right arm and the Bhumisparsha Mudra.
The left hand is placed palm up at sternum, the Buddha Shramana Mudra.

    The Bhumisparsha Mudra is calling the attention to the Truth of the Mudra being presented with it. The Buddha Shramana Mudra is the commitment of the Renunciant. The Renunciant's declaration that "I am an immortal spiritual being, I will live in this world, but I will not be a part of it". It is a recognition of the delusion, stress and suffering caused by the belief in the worldly paradigm and the commitment to not participate in it.

4 - 36   Chi Kung Training Methods
The Mystical Meaning of the Mudra and Movements of Pai He Chuan (continued)

4. The head turns left to gaze into the east.
Left foot steps left into wan-bu turning left to the east,
delivering an overhead cross-block with both fists (Double Dhrithi Mudra).

    The Double Dhrithi Mudra here performed represents the total commitment to the training referred to in the next mudra.

5. *To gaze through the spiritual eye.* The eyes continue to gaze, leveled east.
The weight shifts back to bao-bu (cat stance),
looking through the diamond made by crossing the forearms, holding the tips of the fingers together and bending the wrists backward.

    This mudra is calling our attention to the requirement to train ourselves to consciously maintain our awareness of reality through the spiritual eye. It is through the spiritual eye that our awareness will open up into the experience of Unity, the ultimate reality. When our spiritual awareness becomes fully developed our consciousness will operate solely through the spiritual eye. This training is required to efficiently develop our spiritual awareness. This ability is first developed through the practice of meditation and eventually through all activities.

6. The eyes continue to gaze into the east.
A flying front kick is performed with a wan-bu recovery and a low cross-block (double fists).

    The experience of the opening of the spiritual eye results in an experience of spiritual Joy. The flying kick is an expression of this Joy. The Double Dhrithi Mudra performed with the low cross block, represents the emphatic and total commitment referred to in the spiritual eye training and a reaffirmation of the Joy experienced with the opening of the spiritual eye.

7. The head turns to the right with the gaze leveled west. Pivot on the left back foot turning to the right, the front right foot steps 180 degrees to face west recovering with the right foot in front wan-bu and another low cross-block (Double Dhrithi Mudra).

    This Double Dhrithi Mudra performed with the low cross block again represents the emphatic and total commitment referred to in the spiritual eye training. This second performance in the opposite direction is emphasizing the all encompassing nature of this training.

8. The head turns to the right with the gaze leveled east.
The right foot steps backward into ma-bu (horse stance) to face the north (the stance faces north but the head is turned to the right to face the east),
as a horizontally delivered hammer-fist strike is delivered east (Dhrithi Mudra).

    This Dhrithi Mudra is directed toward the importance of the meaning of the next mudra.

9. The head continues to face the east with the gaze leveled there.
The right fist opens into Abaya Mudra,
the left foot steps east into wan-bu (bow stance) delivering a front crane punch (Dhrithi Mudra).

    The Abaya Mudra is an affirmation of the declaration "I am an Immortal Spiritual Being of Infinite Peace and Fearlessness".

Chi Kung Training Methods
The Mystical Meaning of the Mudra and Movements of Pai He Chuan (continued)

10. The head continues to face the east with the gaze leveled there.
The right foot steps east into wan-bu (bow stance), delivering the Double Abaya Mudra.
    This Double Abaya Mudra is an emphatic emphasis of the previous one handed delivery.

11. The head turns to the left with the gaze leveled north.
The right foot steps east, the body turns north and drops into ma-bu (horse stance) delivering Double Abaya Mudra.
    This Double Abaya Mudra is a dramatic emphasis of the previous two handed delivery.

12. The head continues to face the north with the gaze leveled there.
Double separate into double Buddha-Shramana.
The body rises into shoulder-width ma-bu (horse stance) simultaneous with the drop of the arms crossing and then uncrossing into double Bhumisparsha with the arms downward and parallel.
    The Buddha Shramana Mudra is the commitment of the Renunciant.

13. *Back stance one, with Bhumisparsha and Buddha-shramana.* This sequence of the three back stances became the *Repulse the Monkey* sequence in Tai Chi 108.
(a) The head turns to level the gaze west, the right foot steps east, dropping into ma-bu (horse stance. The arms cross, the left hand reaches to right ear above left arm, right arm reaches diagonally low across the torso, palm up.
(b) Then the feet pivot into ssu lieu-bu stance (back stance),
the arms are pulled apart so that the left arm is parallel to the left leg and left hand into a low bhumisparsha.
The right arm reaches behind the head, 45 degrees at the elbow, into a Buddha-shramana at the height of the top of the head.
    The Bhumisparsha is stating the Truth of the meaning of the Buddha Shramana.

14. *Back stance two, with Bhumisparsha and Buddha-shramana.*
(a) The head continues to look west as the right foot steps forward into the west, into ma-bu. The arms cross, right hand reaches to left ear above right arm, left arm reaches diagonally low across the torso, palm up.
(b) Then the feet pivot into ssu lieu-bu stance, the arms are pulled apart, right arm parallel to the right leg and right hand into a low Bhumisparsha. The left arm reaches behind the head, 45 degrees at the elbow, into a Buddha-shramana at the height of the top of the head.

15. *Back stance three, with Bhumisparsha and Buddha-shramana.*
(a) The head turns to look west again with a 360 degree turn to the left. The left foot steps backward 180 degrees to the west into ma-bu, arms cross left hand reaches to right ear above left arm, right arm reaches diagonally low across the torso palm up.
(b) Then the feet pivot into ssu lieu-bu stance, the arms are pulled apart left arm parallel to the left leg and left hand into a low bhumisparsha. The right arm reaches behind the head, 45 degrees at the elbow, into a Buddha-shramana at the height of the top of the head.

4 - 38 Chi Kung Training Methods
The Mystical Meaning of the Mudra and Movements of Pai He Chuan(continued)

16. The head turns to look the north.
The right foot steps behind the left into a cross stance.
The arms deliver a low cross block with a double Bhumisparsha mudra.

17. The head continues to look north.
The right foot steps east into ma-bu.
The arms deliver a focused double abaya mudra, chest level.

18. The head continues to look north.
Maintain the ma-bu.
The arms deliver the circles of the separate technique and a double Buddha-shramana.

19. The head continues to look north.
The feet are brought together as the body rises into a half ma-bu.
The arms cross, then straighten and drop into a double Bhumisparsha.

20. The head continues to look north.
A Double Dhrithi mudra is performed as the fists are rise to a position just above the hips, palms down.

21. The head continues to face north.
The right knee dips inward twisting the body to the left as the right elbow delivers an inward block north to what was the bodies center line before the twist.

22. The head continues to face north.
The left knee dips inward twisting the body to the right as the left elbow delivers an inward block north to what was the bodies center line before the twist.

23. This movement became *The White Crane Spreads its Wings* in the Tai Chi 108.
(a) The head turns to level the gaze east.
The legs continue the twist pivoting into a cross stance.
The arms rotate and cross, left hand reaches to right ear above left arm, right arm reaches diagonally low across the torso palm up.
(b) Then the left knee rises into a Crane Stance as the arms are pulled apart, left arm parallel to the left thigh and left hand into a low Bhumisparsha Mudra.
The right arm reaches behind the head, 45 degrees at the elbow, into a Buddha-Shramana Mudra at the height of the top of the head.

Chi Kung Training Methods
The Mystical Meaning of the Mudra and Movements of Pai He Chuan (continued)

24. The head continues to look east.
The left hand rises into an Abaya Mudra,
the left leg delivers a front kick east recovering in the east and without a pause in movement,
the right leg steps into the east recovering a wan-bu as the right fist (Dhrithi Mudra) delivers a front crane punch into the east.

    The experience of release from bondage from the belief in the worldly paradigm is replaced with the experience of Infinite Joy that is expressed in the performance of the kick. The experience of release from bondage is expressed in the performance of the Buddha-Shramana Mudra presented in the previous movement *The White Crane Gazes East and Spreads its Wings*. This is the experience of the renunciant when the renunciation is fully realized (when all delusion, stress and suffering disappears from the awareness of the renunciant).

25. *The White Crane Spreads its Wings 2*.
The head turns left and the gaze is leveled into the west.
The right foot steps east into ma-bu.
The arms cross, left hand reaches to right ear above left arm, right arm reaches diagonally low across the torso palm up.
Then the left knee rises into a Crane Stance as the arms are pulled apart, left arm parallel to the left thigh and left hand into a low Bhumisparsha.
The right arm reaches behind the head, 45 degrees at the elbow, into a Buddha-Shramana at the height of the top of the head.

    The Buddha-Shramana is the mudra of the renunciant and the Bhumisparsha expresses the Truth of the associated mudra.

26. The head continues its leveled gaze into the west.
The left hand rises into an Abaya Mudra, the left leg delivers a front kick west recovering ma-bu facing the west.
The right hand delivers Abaya Mudra chest level into the west,
as the left hand performs Varada Mudra in front of and just left of the left hip, facing the east.

    The kick is an expression of the Infinite Joy experienced in the fully realized renunciation presented by the Buddha-Shramana Mudra in the previous movement. The Abaya Mudra is an expression of the best possible intentions. The Varada Mudra is a request for divine assistance in the incorporation of the Five Perfections into one's consciousness. The Five Perfections is an outline of the process used to experience complete spiritual realization that is used within the Shaolin Tradition.

27. The head turns right and the gaze is leveled east. No foot work.
The right hand delivers an Abaya Mudra with a knife hand strike into the east.

28. The head continues its leveled gaze east. No foot work.
The left fist delivers a palm up hammer fist (Dhrithi Mudra) into the palm of the right hand.

4 - 40   Chi Kung Training Methods
The Mystical Meaning of the Mudra and Movements of Pai He Chuan(continued)

29. The gaze continues to leveled east.
No foot work.
The left fist opens and the knuckles of a right Dhrithi Mudra, is placed into the open palm of the left hand (Abaya Mudra).

30. The gaze continues to leveled east.
No foot work.
Then both hands move together to the left hip stopping with the knuckles of the right fist (Dhrithi Mudra) vertical in the open left palm, which presents the Varada Mudra, just left of the left hip. The Varada Mudra in the left hand must face the east.

31. The head turns to the right to face the west.
The left foot steps Southeast into a wan-bu as the body turns to the right to face the West.
As the turn is made the arms reach out in front of the center of the chest.
Rooted in the wan-bu and with the arms straight they continue moving and rising in an arc over the head, then, elbow bending, down to the center of the chest.
Then the arms continue reaching, as the elbows straighten out, again in front of the center of the chest, as the left knee is raised into the crane stance.
The wrist of the right fist is placed horizontal in the "Y" formed by left thumb and index finger, with the palm of the left hand facing West (a version of the Abaya Mudra).

   The Abaya Mudra is an affirmation of the declaration "I am an Immortal Spiritual Being of Infinite Peace and Fearlessness". The right fist is the Dhrithi Mudra affirming the Truth of this declaration. The simultaneous performance of these mudra originate from the center of the chest.

32. The head continues facing west.
The right fist drops to the right hip, palm up.
The left leg delivers a front kick west, recovering in front with a wan-bu.
The right foot then steps west as the right Dhrithi Mudra delivers a front crane punch west.
The left fist (Dhrithi Mudra) is pulled to the left hip as the right crane punch (also a Dhrithi Mudra) is focused with the chi-han "Yi" (chi shout mantra, "Yi" is Chinese for the number one).

   The kick is an expression of Joy. The Dhrithi Mudra, represents the Truth of this expression. The crane punch is delivered with the chi-han "Yi". The chi-han mantra is also used to unify the body, mind and soul into one ultimate commitment. The previous pair of mudra and these two, are being tied together into a supreme focus of the consciousness. The source of the movement of this pair of these double mudra, comes from the center of the chest, the heart. And the entire body's mass (heart, mind and soul) is moving behind the kick and final crane punch (the Dhrithi Mudra). The affirmation and declaration of this multiple combination of mudra and mantra is: "Coming from my heart, mind, and soul, and the mystical experience of my total being, I emphatically state that *I am a Bodhisattva*".

Chi Kung Training Methods
The Mystical Meaning of the Mudra and Movements of Pai He Chuan(continued)

33. The head turns left to face the east.
The body turns left to face the east as the left foot steps to the right foot,
feet together, fists at the sides (a Double Dhrithi Mudra).

34. The form ends as the hands are placed together in front of the chest, with a bow.
   This hand placement is the Namaste Mudra.
The Namaste Mudra is a recognition of Spiritual Unity, "We are One".

The regulation of the **Five Disciplines of Chi Kung** (*wu tiao*) are required for efficient Chi Kung practice. Practice until control becomes natural and automatic (control without control, *wuwei*)

1) The Discipline of Regulating the Body - Tyau Shenn
Correct posture, relaxed, centered, balanced, rooted, coordinated
head suspended makes it possible for Yi (Wisdom Mind) to lead Chi (internal energy)

2) The Discipline of Regulating the Breathing - Tyau Shyi
1) abdominal breathing (post-natal breathing) and a slight contraction and raising of anus
2) reverse abdominal breathing (pre-natal breathing) coordinate the inhale with an inward movement of the lower abdomen and a slight contraction and raising of anus

3) The Discipline of Regulating the Mind - Tyau Hsin
Control the emotional mind (Hsin); eliminate irrational thought process and emotional extremes. Achieve calm, peaceful, focused concentration (Wu Hin), so Yi can lead Chi.

4) The Discipline of Regulating the Chi - Tyau Chi
regulate Chi with total concentration and the application of the will
a) control circulation of Chi (smooth and strong)
b) build-up Chi
c) lead Chi to skin and marrow
d) lead Chi to brain and the Upper Tan Tien (the Spiritual Eye)

5) The Discipline of Regulating the Spirit - Tyau Shen
hold Yi (attention) at the Upper Tan Tien (Spiritual Eye)
achieve Wu Chi consciousness (Buddhahood, Christ Consciousness)

Walking Chi Kung Some key points in the practice of walking chi kung such as Wu Tai Hsing
- Suspend the spine
- Body movement is performed in a chain reaction as in the movement of the snake:
    always started with the feet then moves through the legs
    directed by the waist
    completed with the hands
- Make all movements smooth and natural
- Mind, meditatively concentrated
- The key to advancing from external to internal is in the coordination in the movement of the huiyin/anus and breath; a slight contraction and lift with the inhale, release on the exhale.
- Feel the body as a unit of energy moving in the Infinite Ocean of Energy.
- A relaxed body with the coordination of body, breath, mind and chi is the key to walking chi kung energization: energy accumulation, transportation and balancing.

Chi Kung Training Methods Important Concepts in the Practice of Chi Kung

Levels of Consciousness
The Three Beginner Levels   1) Unconscious 2) Subconscious 3) Waking conscious
The Three Advanced Levels   4) Super conscious 5) Christ conscious 6) Cosmic conscious

Aspects of Consciousness
1) Wisdom Mind (Yi)   2) Emotional Mind (Hsin)   3) the Will (Jyu) the Yi generates Jyu

Energy Sources (The Three Flowers)
1) Essence (Jieng) energy from the physical body   2) Internal Energy (Chi)   3) Spirit (Shen)
"The Three Flowers Bloom at the Top (Upper Tan Tien)" this is the imagery of "Chop with Fist" also the Ishvara Mudra, the opening movements of the hsing Pai She Chuan and the Crane Breath

The Three Fields of Elixir
1) Upper Dan Tien - Spiritual Eye
    Distribution of Chi to the Spiritual Eye stabilizes Yi and firms Shen
2) Middle Dan Tien - Solar Plexus
    Post-birth Chi (Chi from food and air) is processed and gathered here
3) Lower Dan Tien - Naval Center
    Mixes and Stores Pre-birth Chi (chi converted from essence)
    and Post-birth Chi (chi accumulated from external sources, air, food, etc.)

The Three Currents - major paths for energy transportation
1) Fire Path - major Chi circuit of health and vitality
        Governing and Conception Vessels   (small circulation)
2) Wind Path - Yang to Yin balancing of Chi
        Conception Vessel, lower to middle Dan Tien
3) Water Path - mental and spiritual cultivation
        Thrusting Vessel, Huiyin to Upper Dan Tien, through the spinal cord

Triple Burner - Sanjiao
1) Upper Burner - lung, converts air to Chi
2) Middle Burner - stomach, converts food to Chi
3) Lower Burner - lower abdomen, processes Chi

Three Gates of Small Circulation - San Gunn - Generally a persistent application of *will* is required to transport Chi through these cavities on the governing and thrusting vessels.
1) Wie Lu Cavity - tail bone   2) Jar Gi Cavity - heart   3) Yu Gen Cavity - medulla

Three Gates of Chi Exchange
Chi can relatively easily be absorbed or expelled through these cavities
1) Yongquan - Bubbling Well Spring; sole of foot, in the forward area of the arch
2) Laogong - Labor Palace; center of palm of hand
3) Yu Gen - Jade Pillow; medulla, the hollow spot on the neck just bellow the base of the skull

PART V

TRAINING METHODS FOR MARTIAL TECHNIQUE

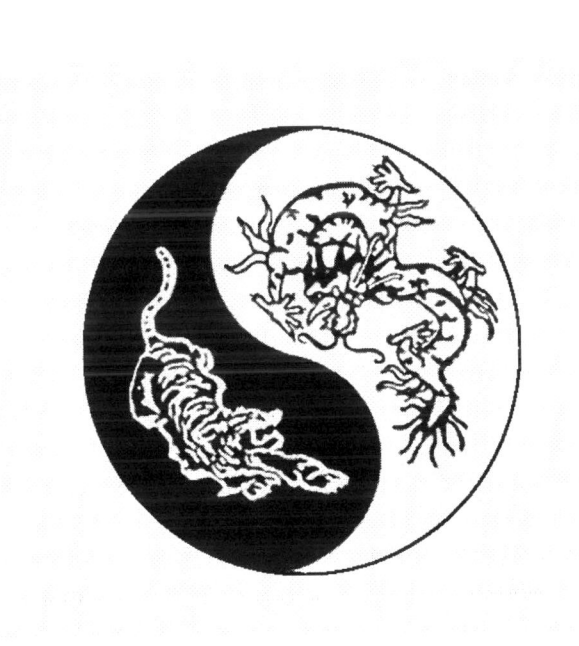

Training Martial Technique

Introduction

The martial training is considered part of the Shaolin Crane System. The Shaolin Crane System is preparatory for the spiritual training. Since the body, mind and soul are interconnected, each one influencing the other two, the physical training is used to enhance mental and spiritual development. The physical stamina that develops from the martial training, influences and transfers to the mental stamina that is needed for the sustained effort required for achieving the goal of self-realization. The mental stimulation required to develop martial ability is very substantial. This stimulation enhances mental ability. The intuition is developed in the selection of: effective techniques, combinations and the performance of movement in the various applications. Concentration, intuition, and meditational ability are synergistically developed by the incorporation of energy accumulation methods into the performance of the movements. These energy accumulation methods are part of the Shaolin Consciousness Energization Process that is used to achieve the goal of spiritual realization. Since the energization methods are part of the Shaolin Snake System there is an over lapping of the Crane and Snake systems within the martial training.

The martial training develops confidence not only in the social arena but internally too. The self-confidence develops slowly, almost imperceptibly; but eventually becomes fearlessness. The effect is a dramatic reduction in stress and stress symptoms which will help remove psychological impediments and make larger amounts of energy available for the spiritual training. The developed self-confidence will make one more effective socially. But the real value of this developed self-confidence is in the fearlessness required to face the sthana and defeat the klesa. Sthana are ego defense mechanisms and the personality masks one wears, socially and internally, to protect oneself from personal insecurities. The sthana are usually subconscious until they are exposed through the process of self examination. Since these sthana are failures to face truth, they are stressful and a substantial energy drain. Klesa are the psychological demons: ignorance, self-centeredness, and fear and all their manifestations (hatred, greed, jealousy, procrastination, etc.). The ego can be the most daunting of adversaries. But with the defeat of the klesa, required steps on the path to spiritual perception will have been taken.

The Shaolin Crane System includes training in the classic forms, combat forms, technique combination drills, the martial technique and application drills.

Within this chapter are some pertinent details the beginning and advanced Shaolin Monk must have of martial arts knowledge.

The Tao Te Ching - Lao Tsu

"The most skillful warriors are not warlike; the best fighters are not wrathful; the mightiest conquerors never strive; the greatest masters are ever lowly.
 This is the glory of non-strife; and the might of utilization; those equal heaven, they were the goal of the ancients."

Martial Technique Training — Temple Hsing (DVDs available, see page D-1)

Temple Hsing (monk forms)   The nine temple hsing specifically used for monk training are:
1) San Zan Chuan
2) Sei San Chuan
3) San Sei Chuan
4) Wu Tai Hsing
5) Wu Shi Si
6) Wu Hsing Chuan
7) Pai He Chuan
8) Pai He No Kon
9) Pai She Chuan
10) Bodhisattva Tao

According to the oral tradition, three of these hsing are the original used by Bodhidharma to teach his first monks at the original Shaolin Temple. They are San Zan Chuan, Sei San Chuan, and San Sei Chuan. These three hsing are said to have come from the Vajramukti yoga sect in India. The remaining seven all have Shaolin origins.

The hsing training has several purposes specifically aimed at developing spiritual awareness. These are:
- develop physical strength for the stamina required for meditation.
- enhance mental abilities to comprehend concepts, techniques and methods used to develop spiritual awareness.
- raise energy levels to develop the intuition, to enhance the results of meditation.
- teach spiritual concepts, through the mudra within the hsing, to speed up the process of developing spiritual awareness.
- build and sustain motivational levels so that the results of the training can be realized.
- Samasthana: samasthana is self examination/self awareness training used to expose the sthana to the self. The sthana is the personality; its belief system (including its limitations, delusions and illusions) and the resulting thought, habits and behavior patterns. This is the first step in the Personality Purification Process required for Spiritual Realization.

Martial abilities developed through forms practice are:
precision of movement   timing   strength   coordination   balance
proprioceptive ability   agility   speed   stamina

Mental abilities developed through the practice of forms which can make one more efficient at whatever one does and are prerequisite to the development of spiritual awareness are:
Wu Hsin   self confidence   discipline   perseverance   concentration
will   memory enhancement   discernment   determination   intuition

Classic Hsing

At first glance the practice of classic Hsing does not appear to be an objective approach to the practice and development of fighting ability. And what possible benefit to spiritual awareness could fighting ability be? The first thing that hits you as one watches the performance of classic forms is that the stance is not conducive to defense against punches and kicks. The back is held straight exposing the front of the torso. The chin is held up exposing not only the chin, but also the throat, nose and the eyes. The torso is held almost square to the direction one faces, which very effectively exposes the abdomen and chest.

Martial Technique Training   **Classic Hsing** - (continued)

Since the body's weight tends to be held forward, it will take more time to move backward when that movement is called for. The back leg is held too straight for efficient mobility. The front foot and knee point straight forward exposing the groin. The back fist is many times held on the hip; the wrong place if one wishes to defend against any kind of attack. According to basic learning theory one must duplicate, as closely as possible, the activity that is being learned. But in forms practice there is no partner to interact with. Without a partner you can not learn to obtain range for your techniques or learn to defend against anything. Combat obviously involves at least two people. Don't give up on forms practice yet though; this will make perfect sense once the reasons are explained.

There are several reasons for the illogical stance in classic forms. The first involves responsibility on the part of the teacher to teach fighting skills only to people who are worthy of true instruction. There is a moral problem with teaching fighting skills to those that would use them for inappropriate purposes. Traditionally, forms training was the primary method of teaching the arts. So the beginning students were not really taught to fight until they had proven themselves. Since this stance is ridiculous for fighting purposes, people of dubious moral character will not have the patience or trust required to obtain long term results.

But even though the training looks worthless at first glance, the new students are being taught the fundamentals of martial movement and the prerequisite abilities needed to efficiently achieve "perfection". Those whose personalities have evolved appropriately find that the most effective techniques and fighting strategies are hidden within the forms to the extent that they can only be discovered when the form is mastered (which takes at least many months of practice). The precise placement and movement of the appendages and posture teach discipline, discernment and proprioceptive awareness (the ability to know exactly where one's body parts are without looking at them). Movement from one precise placement to another develops precision of movement. These abilities are required to achieve maximum efficiency in martial movement. Once the forms are mastered the practice of forms will further develop the other physical abilities required such as coordination, timing, speed, balance, strength, stamina and agility. The classic posture of the stance is used to keep the mind in an alert state to enhance the intuitional ability and the energy collection methods used during the performance of the forms.

Even though at first glance prearranged sequences of movement seem like they could not possibly teach spontaneity of movement, yet, they in fact do. Bruce Lee made a big issue out of what he perceived as fact, that the practice of prearranged technique sequences does not replicate the spontaneity of combat and for this reason advised against the practice of forms. But apparently Bruce lacked the patience required to discover the awesome benefits that can be obtained from this practice. The movements of the sequences are committed to memory and performed without any fore brain activity; without telling yourself to move this way or that. This is called "wu hsin" (chinese) mu shin (japanese) and translates as no-mindedness. Wu hsin is required for efficient self defense ability and any creative act (thought or movement). It is also a component of every intuitive experience and therefore a requirement for true meditation (concentration used to experience the Infinite).

Wu Hsin in Forms Training

The awareness must be externalized throughout form performance to achieve optimum balance and efficiency while moving. Internalized attention will distract and limit the awareness from the totality of the experience. It will dramatically limit the ability to learn what can be gained from forms training. In combat, an internalized awareness will leave one very vulnerable. Internalizing awareness takes place when the attention is isolated to specific aspects of a task or using words in thought processes. Forms practice is exercise in maintaining the totality of the experience and opening it up to all possibilities. Opening up the awareness to the totality of the experience is wu hsin. Wu hsin is accomplished by doing the task without using words in the thought processes of doing. The use of words in thought processes slows thought down and limits the thoughts to only the words that you know. When thinking without words, the awareness can open up to the use of intuition. When using intuition the awareness has the potential to access anything and everything. In combat this can enable the awareness to know the intentions of another person and what they are going to do next. It can also make you aware of the most appropriate thing for you to do next. In forms practice it will allow the recognition: of stance efficiency, efficiency in movement, efficiency in the delivery of energy, of all the different ways the movements can be used and much more. In meditation, intuition will not operate efficiently without opening up the awareness to the totality of every possibility. The awareness can not even get a glimpse of Spirit without it. It is wu hsin that makes the efficient use of intuition and the externalization of the mind possible. The use of wu hsin requires training and self-mastery. Forms practice is wu hsin and self mastery training. With the required mental application and daily practice, the forms training can become meditation in movement.

In order to do well at anything one must be able to concentrate on what is being attended to. The more focused the concentration, the better the results. *Kime* is completely focused concentration. When kime is accomplished as the forms are practiced, the ability to concentrate can be exercised and developed. The ability to concentrate transfers to whatever one attempts and is prerequisite for meditation.

A level gaze will assist in holding one's attention on the task at hand. A lowered gaze has the tendency of scattering the thoughts. A raised gaze will move one out of the physical arena into the realm of pure thought. We lower our gaze when we fall asleep and raise our gaze when we meditate. In forms practice, with few exceptions, the gaze is held level, with mind operating in a state of wu hsin.

Just to learn forms requires a considerable amount of practice. But the real benefits are obtained over long term training, after the form(s) are learned and can be performed in the mental state of *wu hsin*.

Forms practice teach breath control, one of the five disciplines of chi kung. The coordination of movement and focus of the breath will increase power of technique. Breath control can invigorate the body by oxygenating blood and body tissue. Advanced breath control techniques can super-energize the body and consciousness, enabling optimum health, enhancement of mental ability and increasing spiritual awareness.

Kiai is an explosive shout used to mobilize physical and internal energy. Many forms present opportunities to practice this technique.

The practice of forms can teach external and internal energy application, (accumulation, conservation and transportation of chi) which is required for technique power and the Energization of Consciousness.

Forms practice is a performance art which has great visual beauty. The beauty of the performance of forms can be appreciated by the performer and the spectator.

There are many, many hours when one can practice but does not have a partner available. Forms practice is available for these times. But in addition to this reason for forms training, forms have training value of their own, unfathomable to a beginner. Repetition of forms practice, with intense self-application, will hone the will. It will instill the fortitude and determination required to stay on task until the goal is reached.

Forms have value as a catalog of technique and fighting strategies of a fighting style. Although the techniques as performed in most classic forms are not intended to be used in a real self defense situation. Woven into the sequences of movement within the classic forms are advanced fighting strategies and technique, making each of them a text book of martial information. The forms are a catalog of spiritual concepts, fighting strategies and technique that continue to make available to us this information that may otherwise have been forgotten.

The classic forms have great historical value. As these forms are mastered it is possible to understand the motivation, experience and knowledge of the Shaolin Masters who created them. Through the practice of forms it is possible to know the thoughts of the masters who created and developed the Shaolin Tradition; not only gaining historical knowledge but also insights into the "Way".

Martial Technique Training

Training Martial Technique

Although some general rules of fighting strategies can be outlined, there are no absolute right or wrong rules for fighting strategies because no situation is exactly the same. There is always a situation that requires an exception. But every detail of movement and posture must have a legitimate reason in order to make one's ability the best that it can be. The pertinent details of each situation must be perceived to be efficiently responded to. The development of abilities in mental alertness, objectivity, analysis, discernment, cause and effect, are emphasized. Additional skills that are required are: martial knowledge, determination, concentration, self confidence, courage, discipline, efficient spontaneity, wu-hsin and intuition; all of which are trained and developed in the practice of combat training. The abilities developed in learning to adapt efficiently to every situation will transfer to everything that one attempts. The combat training will develop mental abilities and habits of thought that will be used throughout ones life, for everything one thinks and does.

Abilities required to efficiently respond to physical situations are: speed & quickness, timing, coordination, stamina, strength, proprioceptive sense, agility, flexibility, balance, precision.

In addition to self-defense ability, a very high level of physical fitness will develop enabling the body to process much larger amounts of energy that can be used to enhance meditation ability.

The exercises, drills and advice outlined in the next few pages will be of some assistance in training each of these abilities.

Soft versus Hard

The concepts of soft and hard usually refer to methods of fighting. The hard methods of fighting emphasize very direct offensive and defensive technique. These are characterized by linear and force against force techniques. Examples are punches and kicks launched from a stationary position or moving straight toward the target as the technique is launched. Hard blocks are those that meet an incoming attack head on or at a ninety degree angle. In many instances hard blocks are delivered in a way to damage the attacking appendage. The soft methods of fighting emphasize offensive and defensive technique that are delivered from angles other than from the original straight in position. This can dramatically increase the number of target areas available. These techniques many times rely on body movement and footwork to set up the angles for the delivery. Soft defensive techniques are characterized by deflection and redirection of incoming attacks thereby neutralizing the attacks and exposing targets for counters. These also may be applied in a way to injure the attacker at the same time.

Martial Technique Training (continued)

Stance, Posture

If the length of the foot placement is too long, mobility will be impeded. If the length is too short, balance will be disturbed. As with almost everything, a medium is most often the best option. Adhere to the Rule of No Extremes.

Both knees are held bent so that one is able to most efficiently use the thigh muscles for mobility. The center of gravity is lowered, again, making mobility more efficient but also enhancing balance.

The front knee and thigh is usually used to make the groin harder to hit. This is accomplished by keeping both knees bent and turning the front foot and knee in 45 degrees. Since the front knee and thigh end up in front of the groin, it is harder to attack.

The back foot is usually used to stabilize the stance and for this reason it is usually placed almost a shoulders width to its side of the front foot.

In order to make most efficient use of the muscles in the calf for mobility, the back foot is placed pointing 45 degrees out from direction one is facing.

For optimum mobility, the weight is held evenly on both feet in a fighting stance. In a situation in which one does not know which direction one must go next, the distance and time will be greater if one must move into the direction of the foot that has less weight. Distance and time are critical in a fighting situation.

In most cases the torso should be held on a diagonal to the attacker. This will limit the area of the torso that can be hit easily, since the entire front of the torso will not be facing the attacker. Also, if the shoulders are held on a 45 degree angle to the target, both sides of the body will be in a cocked position. This means that neither the hands, feet, hips or shoulders will have to be drawn back (called a wind-up) to generate power for offensive technique.

Any movement preliminary to an attack, can give the intention away making it easier to defend against. These preliminary movements are called **telegraphing**.

A wind-up is ok if one has the time. But in most cases the time element is too crucial for the use of a wind-up. The wind-up should be accomplished in the stance and posture.

If the head is tilted forward, the jaw, nose and eyes will be harder to hit.

The jaw will be able to take greater impacts if the mouth is kept shut with the teeth together.

Martial Technique Training - (continued)

Eye Position and Gaze

If the gaze is focused on the attacker's hands, it will be hard to see a foot coming; if focused on the feet it will be hard to see a hand coming. One should look toward the center of the torso without focusing the gaze. Develop peripheral vision to take in the whole. Since this spot is the location of the center of weight, movement many times begins here, allowing the earliest physical detection of intention and attack.

Hands and Hand Position

Hands, forearms and elbows are used both offensively and defensively. Depending on the situation the hands can be held open or closed, or either one hand open and the other closed.

If a hand is held open the fingers and thumb should be held tightly together. The reason being that the fingers will be less likely to be injured if they are held together. The fingers are stronger together than when they are apart.

Generally, at least one hand should be held high to protect the head; both hands if the attacker is a headhunter.

Technique Power

Technique power is developed by efficiently involving as many muscle cells of each muscle used as possible and as many muscle groups as possible. This is called external power.

Internal power is generated through mental control of chi. This mental control arises from developed abilities of concentration and will power.

Technique power usually begins at the back foot and is generated by muscles contracting in a chain reaction through the body to and usually *through* the striking surface (target).

After maximum involvement of muscle groups, speed of delivery may be the most important factor in technique power and efficiency, since speed (velocity) is the most influencing variable. The physics of energy delivery is; "energy = mass x velocity x velocity".

Not only is speed important for the delivery of energy, but the faster the technique is, the harder it is to defend against it.

The body's mass is pretty much a constant. But in order to use it efficiently, one must be able to put it into motion with the technique being delivered, and *line it up* behind the weapon (fist, foot, etc.).

Martial Technique Training - (continued)

Hand Techniques

Do not underestimate the need for good wrist and finger strength for the delivery of hand techniques. The power of a technique depends on the strength of the weapon delivering it.

Grabs are a very versatile offensive technique. They can be used to attack: pressure points, soft flesh, joints, bones. They can also be used to set up targets, to control striking attacks coming in, to take control of attackers and to deliver throws. Grabbing techniques deserve considerable exploration.

An open hand is most easily used defensively.

Palm blocks can efficiently be turned offensive with an edge of hand strike.

In order to develop full efficiency with the back knuckle strike, the wrist is used to snap the technique into its focus like a whip. The common error is to keep the wrist rigid, and strike with the forearm and fist as if it were a club.

As punching techniques are delivered it is important that the elbow be directly behind the fist as it is delivered and focused. If the elbow is not directly behind the fist, the energy of the punch will dissipate as the elbow deflects to the side of the fist during impact.

When delivering front punches, hook punches and upper cuts, it is important to keep the wrist straight. On impact, when the wrist is bent, the wrist will have a tendency to bend even more. This will cause power loss and possibly injury to the wrist.

Kicking Techniques

The complete bending of the knee is required for developing maximum kicking power (with the exception of the crescent type kicks).

When delivering front kicks or roundhouse kicks, the knee must point at the target as the kick is delivered. If this is not done the kick will miss its mark or it will lack the power it could have had.

Since the quadriceps and gluteus maximus are the largest and most powerful muscles in the human body, the side and back kicks have the definite potential of being your most powerful kicks. To most efficiently use these muscles and obtain full power when delivering these kicks, the knee must be bent completely and the knee pulled up in front of the body to chamber the hip before delivery.

To line the body up behind side and back kicks for efficient power delivery, the heel must travel in a straight line to the target; in a thrusting motion. "Chamber the hip, then fire the heel."

Martial Technique Training - (continued)
Fighting Strategies

The concept of opening doors and windows must be thoroughly understood in order to get through a good defense, and to develop one. Doors are positions of the feet and legs that make one vulnerable to attack. Windows are positions of hands and arms that make one vulnerable to attack. Much experimentation with this concept is required to obtain proficiency.

At novice levels it is easier to respond to a punching attack with a kick. And it is easier to respond to a kicking attack with a punch. "Kick a puncher and punch a kicker." This strategy will smooth out your counters and make them more effective.

Be able to strike or kick with either hand or either foot.
"The less limited you are, the more efficient you will be."

When countering, it is safer to step to the attackers back side than to remain in front of him. The position in front of him exposes you to his back hand and foot. For this reason it is a good idea to develop an arsenal of efficient counters that can be used moving out of range of his reverse techniques and staying in range for yours. One of the corner stones of the Yue Chia system is this side stepping strategy.

The ability to use mobility in side stepping attacks is a definite advantage, but do not neglect the duck and the slip.

There are situations when the most efficient counter is to back up. There are times when the most efficient offensive move is straight in. To be efficient, you must train for every situation.

When dealing with multiple attackers, a strategy that must be developed is to counter and move so that one attacker is between you and the other attacker or attackers. The advantage of this strategy is that you will only have to deal with one at a time. Two or more at a time may very well get difficult, very fast.

For real self-defense purposes high kicks are not recommended. Since the foot must travel a greater distance (from the ground to the higher target area) it is easier to detect than a technique that does not travel as far. Easier detection means easier to defend against and easier to counter. Also, with the foot and leg so high in the air, it places one in an unstable position. A position that can be readily taken advantage of.

High kicks do have a place for training purposes. It is probably healthy for the body to exercise the flexibility required for these kicks; as long it is not taken to an extreme. Also, it is necessary to learn how to defend against this type of kick. It would be hard to help your friends learn this necessary ability if one can not deliver high kicks for them.
There are times when a little "flash" may be called for.

Martial Technique Training - (continued)

Mobility

Unnecessary muscle tension will slow one down, interfere with coordination and strip technique of power. It probably is the most common mistake made by martial artists.

Since optimum mobility depends so much on stance, many of the strategies for mobility are the same as the ones recommended for stance training.

Good balance is a requirement for good mobility. Although a long stance may offer greater stability, if the length of the foot placement is too long, mobility will be impeded. If the length is too short, balance will be disturbed.

Both knees are held visibly bent, over the toes, for three reasons: 1) with the knees bent the center of gravity is lowered, thereby enhancing balance and the ability to move 2) the thigh muscles can be used more efficiently for mobility when the knees are sufficiently bent 3) if one drops by bending the knees to more efficiently move at the time of attack or defense, it will slow one down and telegraph intention. In a fighting stance one should be able to jump into the air with power, without having to bend the knees before jumping.

In order to make most efficient use of the muscles in the calf for mobility, the back foot is placed pointing 45 degrees out from the direction one is facing. The common mistake is pointing it to the side or back.

For optimum mobility from a fighting stance, the weight is held evenly on both feet. In a situation in which one does not know which direction one must go next, the distance and time will be greater if one must move into the direction of the foot that has less weight. Distance and time are critical in a fighting situation.

Do not allow the center to rise as one moves. "Stay low as you step." The rising will slow one up and make one less stable.

Cross stepping can put one in a disadvantageous position, especially when dealing with only one person. But, cross stepping can be used to advantage when performing fighting strategies dealing with multiple attackers. The practice of cross stepping in technique drills will develop agility.

To understand martial mobility, develop efficiency with stepping patterns using appropriate technique combinations in the stepping patterns from the List of Yue Chia Stepping Patterns. (See page 5 - 14)

5 - 12   Martial Technique Training - (continued)   Training Tips

It is imperative that the intensity of training be developed gradually. It takes time for the body to adapt to physical stress. Over zealousness will result in injuries that will dramatically slow progress.

Before practice begins one must prepare the body for the activity. Cardiovascular training levels should be reached gradually and the muscles, tendons and joints should be stretched adequately prior to formal training. If this physical preparation is not accomplished training results will be inadequate and the possibility of injury significant.

Whenever practicing self defense techniques, one should begin in a posture that would be held when attacked or attacking, so that the practice movements will be the same as those used in a real application. This practice method will substantially improve one's ability to use the technique.

Always recover from a technique drill with a fighting stance. This habit will prepare one to efficiently handle the development of any situation. One will be less likely to be caught by surprise.   "It is not over until you recover."

It is much easier to learn technique by moving through them slowly at first, than to try to begin learning at fighting speed. By moving through them slowly the correct coordination, precision and timing can be felt much easier, thereby reducing the development of bad habits.

The flexibility required for efficient technique delivery must be trained. This requires daily flexibility drills. Leg swings and leg extensions that mimic kick delivery are highly recommended.

The skill of self examination and objectivity is developed by constant analysis of ones performance (stance, movement, strategies, etc.) for efficiency.

As one practices technique drills and forms the <u>gaze must be focused</u> on the area of the target and the area the incoming weapons would be in. This is crucial for several reasons.
- Without physical focus technique power will be low. Physical focus requires mental focus. Mental focus is facilitated by the visual gaze. It is difficult to obtain physical focus of the technique without the visual focus. During practice "the mind is focused with the gaze of the eyes."
- Without the practice of delivering technique with power, it will be hard to deliver the power when it is really needed.
- When power is low, the workout will not have the exercise potential it would have had if the techniques were delivered with power.
- It is very difficult to develop technique accuracy without the visual gaze. "It is hard to hit what you can not see."
- Without mental focus, movement will tend to be uncoordinated and the recovery will tend to be unbalanced. Visual focus will assist mental focus.

Martial Technique Training - (continued)
Basic Taolu Technique List   (DVD available see page D - 1)

Blocks and Deflections

- front hand and rear hand - left and right delivery, upper and lower levels
- front and rear hand blocks must be demonstrated with palm, fist, hand edge and grab.
- rising wrist block - front hand and rear hand
- glancing arm block - front arm and rear arm

Strikes

- front hand punch (jab) also known as (straight punch) with vertical fist delivery
- rear hand punch (cross) also known as (reverse punch) with vertical fist delivery
- back knuckle strike
- hammer fist strike
    - overhead delivery
    - horizontal delivery
    - rising to rear delivery
- edge of hand strike
    - overhead delivery
    - reverse delivery
    - horizontal from rear hand
- hook punch with horizontal delivery
    - front hand and rear hand
- upper-cut punch
    - front hand and rear hand
- elbow
    - front hand and rear hand
    - forward, reverse, upward and downward deliveries

Kicks

- front kick - front and back leg
- side kick - front and back leg
- roundhouse kick - front and back leg
- back kick - front and back leg
- knee kick - (both rising and roundhouse deliveries), front and back leg
- stomp kick - front and back leg

* All blocking, deflecting, striking and kicking surfaces must be identified.
* Efficiency should be obtained with all techniques and footwork on both sides of the body.
* All sanshou (techniques and combinations) must be accompanied with bufa (foot work).

Martial Technique Training - (continued)

Develop efficiency with stepping patterns using appropriate technique combinations in the stepping patterns from the List of Yue Chia Stepping Patterns.

The List of Yue Chia Stepping Patterns

- Forward step, front foot *
- Backward step, back foot *
- Side step, front foot *
- Side step, back foot *
- Forward side step, front foot *
- Forward side step, back foot *
- Backward side step, front foot *
- Backward side step, back foot *
- Forward diagonal step, front foot *
- Forward diagonal step, back foot *
- Backward diagonal step, front foot *
- Backward diagonal step, back foot *
- Forward cross step, front foot *
- Forward cross step, back foot *
- Backward cross step, front foot *
- Backward cross step, back foot *
- Full forward step, back foot *
- Forward half step, back foot *
- Full backward step, front foot *
- Backward half step, front foot *
- Forward cross step, front foot*
- Cross step, back foot*

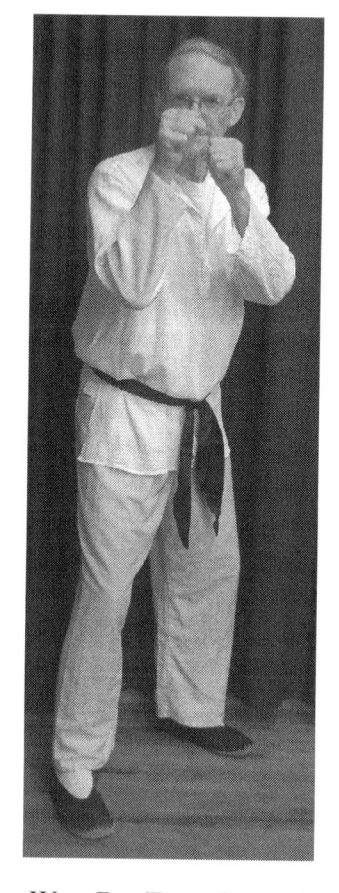

* second foot always steps into placement
    with a recovery position and stance

Wan Bu (Bow Stance)
All stepping patterns begin and recover with this stance

Wan Bu (Bow Stance) description (for more info see page 5 - 7)

Length of the stride should be about a normal walking distance,
feet should be about six inches apart, knees bent and held over the toes,
arms in guard position: fists in front of the face, elbows down, chin dropped behind fists,
torso held front facing 45°, with the front foot's shoulder in front,
the bodies weight is held: evenly on both feet, forward on the feet, but the heels on the floor

Martial Technique Training **Wu Hsing Chuan**

Wu Hsing Chuan - The Form of the Ancient Wisdom of the Five Animals
    The form, techniques and combinations   (DVD available see page D-1)
    This form is not classical and is combat oriented.
    It should eventually be performed with its mirror image, as one form.

Key   R   right   E   east   S   south   NW   northwest   SE   southeast
         L   left   W   west   N   north   SW   southwest

1) The Opening Begins, facing E with a bow, feet and hands together.
L foot steps forward into a Cat Stance and Dragon Mudra.
R foot steps forward into a Bow Stance and the Tiger Claw Mudra.
R knee comes up into a Crane Stance and Crane posture.
R foot steps back into a Bow Stance and the L hand delivers White Snake Puts Out Tongue.
The weight shifts back into a Cat Stance and the Panther Hand Posture.
R foot steps back, feet and hands together, Bow.

2) The Dragon combination begins, facing E.
L foot steps apart shoulder width and the hands drop to the sides. 360 degree spin to the R on the R foot. Land with feet shoulder width apart simultaneously delivering straight punches, L to the North and R to the South.
Flying roundhouse kick R leg, then spinning back kick with L. Setting the kick down SE turn 180 degrees to the R to face West, the R foot stepping NW into a long bow stance.

3) The Tiger combination begins, facing W.
As West is faced the R foot steps diagonally to the NW and the L hand blocks and grabs SW.
L roundhouse kick and Tiger Claw face grab R hand.
R roundhouse kick, stomp with same foot with recovery into the Crane stance facing S.

4) The Crane combination begins, facing S.
As the R foot lands with the recovery, turn to the S, simultaneously: 1) lifting the L knee,
2) R hand rises in front of the face and drops palm down at belt level,
3) The L hand from belt level rises to just above eye level directly above the R hand in the White Crane Spreads its Wings posture.
L groin kick with instep, without setting the L foot down deliver the L front kick to abdomen, then with the R leg deliver a flying front kick. Land in a R Bow Stance facing S.

5) The Snake Combination begins, facing S.
The head turns 180 degrees L to face N, deliver a rising hammer fist strike to the rear with the L fist. Then the hands are placed on the floor with the R hand between the legs,
perform a 180 degree leg sweep to the R with the R leg.
As the sweep is completed the R knee comes up and the L knee goes to the floor, as the L fist delivers a downward punch to the floor, with the L knee on the floor the stance faces N.
R foot steps back into a L Bow Stance and the L hand delivers White Snake Puts Out Tongue.

Martial Technique Training   **Wu Hsing Chuan** - (continued)

6) The Panther Combination Begins, facing E.
The R foot leaps E into a R Bow Stance, as a R front punch is delivered. Followed by a L panther punch. R foot steps back, L hand sweeps heel, as you rise and push with the R palm. R foot travels forward with stomp and returns behind to recover a cat stance with the panther posture, facing E.

7) The Close Begins facing E.
L foot steps back to shoulder width apart, hands drop to the sides.
The R foot steps to the L, feet together, hands rise to together, then bow.
R foot steps forward into a Cat Stance and Dragon Mudra.
L foot steps forward into a Bow Stance and the Tiger Claw Mudra.
L knee comes up into a Crane Stance and Crane posture.
L foot steps back into a Bow Stance and R hand performs White Snake Puts Out Tongue.
The weight shifts back into a Cat Stance and the Panther Hand Posture.
L foot steps back, feet and hands together, Bow.

East

Numbers correlate to combinations

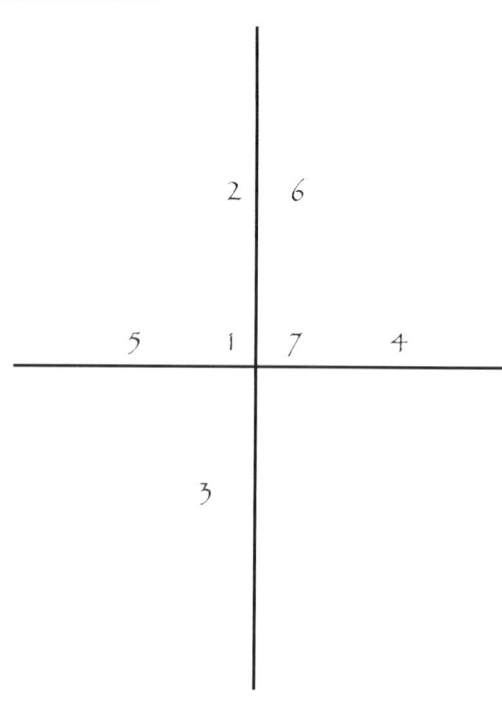

```
              |
              |
           2  | 6
              |
    5     1   | 7      4
   ───────────┼──────────────
              |
           3  |
              |
              |
```

PART VI

REQUIREMENTS FOR MONASTIC TRAINING

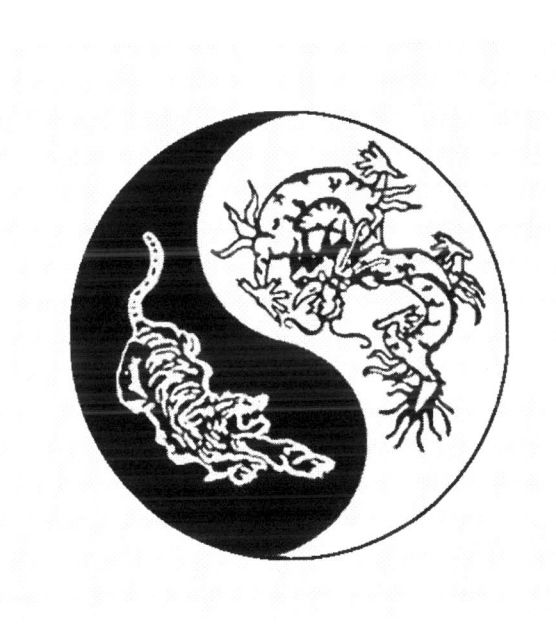

Requirements for Monk Training
Application for Acceptance as a Monk of the Shaolin Temple

Participation as a monk of the Shaolin Order is for those of the Shaolin Brotherhood who wish to make a more meaningful commitment to self-development, the perpetuation of the Shaolin Tradition, and have a greater influence on the positive spiritual evolution of humanity.

Since the Shaolin Tradition was created from a synthesis of many religious and philosophical traditions, a Shaolin Monk must recognize the Truth at the core of all the great religions of the world, and be willing to use constructive information from any source. Also, a Shaolin Monk is not bound to practice only the Shaolin Tradition and **may** at the same time practice another tradition or religion.

The Shaolin Monk must:

- make a commitment to be as efficient as possible in one's efforts toward personal growth and spiritual realization. This is part of the vow the monk must take with the initiation ceremony.

- to train at the Temple at least twice a week, if living within commute distance.

- to live in accord with the moral codes and discipline prescribed by the great religions of the world

- meditate at least twice a day

- obtain the Monk initiation and comply with the vows required by the initiation

- help provide support for the Temple

- invite others to our order who may find some benefit from participation in the activities of the Shaolin Tradition

- be recommended by a Shaolin Monk, and (or) an interview by the Director

- submit a written application to the Director

- follow all of the Temple rules as required of the laity and the order

Application for acceptance in the Shaolin Monastic Order of Michigan, must be made to the Director of the Shaolin Temple of Michigan.

An application for monk training can be found in the appendix page A - 2.

Monastic Levels

Monastic levels are obtained by: meeting the requirements of monkhood, passing the tests of the levels and by meeting any additional requirements as determined by the Director.

Traditional monastic levels within the Shaolin Order are:
1) student 2) disciple 3) monk 4) priest

Uniform requirements of the monastics within the Shaolin Sangha (order of monks).

The student monk may wear the standard white do-gi and belt or sash of the grade color of the corresponding laity level. An option available to the student monk is the white kung-fu uniform with white trim and sash or belt of the grade color of the of the laity level.

The disciple monk may wear any uniform of the previous level and at his or her option the blue kung-fu uniform and (or) sash.

The full monk may wear any uniform of the previous levels and at his or her option a yellow top.

The priest may wear any uniform of the previous levels and may officiate within the Temple wearing the traditional yellow robes of the Shaolin Priest.

A monk of any level may wear the emblem of the Temple on any personal clothing or any uniform.

Reading List:

The Zen Teaching of Bodhidharma: Translated by Red Pine   ISBN 0-86547-399-4
Autobiography of a Yogi: Paramahansa Yogananda, ISBN 0-87612-079-6
Life Surrendered in God: Roy Davis   ISBN 0-87707-246-9
The Eternal Way The Bagavad Gita and Commentary: Roy Davis
A Master Guide to Meditation: Roy Davis   ISBN 0-87707-238-8
Seven Lessons in Conscious Living: Roy Davis   ISBN 0-87707-280-9
The Root of Chinese Qigong: Dr. Yang, Jwing-Ming   ISBN-13: 978-1-886969-50-6
A New Earth, Awakening to Your Life's Purpose: Eckhart Tolle ISBN 978-0-452-28996-3
Change Your Thoughts- Change Your Life: Dr. Wayne W. Dyer   ISBN 978-1-4019-1184-3
Reinventing the Body, Resurrecting the Soul: Deepak Chopra   ISBN 978-0-307-45298-6
The Bodhisattva Warriors: Shifu Nagaboshi Tomio   ISBN 0-87728-785-6

Requirements for Monk Training **The Monk's Vow**

In order to have a long, happy and healthy life that is filled with Joy, a student of the Shaolin Tradition, will incorporate into their life the Five Perfections, the Five Restraints, the Five Observances, and the Five Daily Practices. This will facilitate a direct experience of Spirit in all its aspects.

A personal awareness of Spirit will assist in the spiritual evolution of humanity; moving humanity toward peace and harmony with each other, the Earth and Spirit.

This Vow should be reaffirmed before one goes to sleep and every time one rise from sleep.

The Monk's Vow

I will remove evil from my life with the Five Restraints:
    1) non violence   2) truthfulness   3) non stealing
        4) sensual control   5) non possessiveness

I will cultivate virtue by incorporating into my life the Five Observances:
    1) purity   2) contentment   3) spiritual exercise
        4) self examination/ purification   5) spiritual communion.

I will instill within my consciousness the Five Perfections:
    1) Perfect Compassion and Perfect Charity
    2) Perfect Love and Perfect Morality
    3) Perfect Determination and Perfect Patience
    4) Perfect Discipline and Perfect Effort
    5) Perfect Meditation and Perfect Illumination

I will assist in the liberation of all beings with the Five Daily Practices:
    1) service   2) self purification   3) spiritual study
        4) meditation & prayer and   5) surrender to God.

Through an exercise of my will and through the grace of God, I will bring into my life the complete awareness of Spirit in all its aspects:

    Love, Light, Unity, Compassion, Truth, Wisdom, Joy, Peace, and Bliss.

Requirements for Monk Training — Ceremony Purpose and Outline of Method

Purpose of Ceremony: to make needed changes in our spiritual awareness and circumstances.

Outline and Components of Ceremony

- Self purification - meditation

- Area purification - 1) affirmation and/or prayer*, 2) and/or Staff Ritual, 3) incense

- Energizing of consciousness - chi kung practice

- Creating the sacred sphere (optional, indoors or out) - Staff Ritual

- The Invocation - affirmation and / or prayer*

- The ritual observance - (optional) affirmation and/or prayer*

- Change sought - (optional) affirmation and/or prayer*

- Acknowledgment and Thanking of Spirit - prayer* and/or affirmation

- Dispersing the sacred sphere (optional, indoors or out) - Staff Ritual

Three phases of spiritual realization and ceremony intent

1) Purification: removal of inappropriate conditionings from the personality
   Energization of Consciousness: through prayer*, meditation, chi kung and or chanting

2) Expansion: experiencing the self beyond the body
   The awareness experiences Self Realization

3) Identification: experiencing God in omnipresence (Unity)
   The awareness experiences Christ Consciousness
   and then Cosmic Consciousness

* (All prayer must recognize Unity)

Requirements for Monk Training — Prayer 6-5

Instructions for Prayer

The power of prayer is dramatically enhanced if it delivered from the perspective of Spirit, as Spirit, within Spirit or within an aspect of Spirit. Prayers said to an external being propagate the belief of separateness as opposed to Unity awareness (this can be very counter productive). It is very important to cultivate Unity awareness.

- Prayers can be said audibly or mentally.
- Do not recite prayers absentmindedly. The power and effectiveness of absentmindedly recited prayers is very limited.
- Prayer performance must be delivered **mindfully with fully focused attention and an act of the will.**
- Alert body posture and the Frontal Gaze are mandatory.

Prayers and Affirmations

Opening Prayer for Meditation, Chi Kung or Physical Training

I face the east and I align myself with the Divine Ultimate All .
I bow to thee, Oh Great Spirit, that pervades the universe and beyond.
Whose movement has given rise to the Yin and the Yang, the Father and Mother of all.
Whose creative vibrating energy has begotten the five elements
and the one thousand and one things.
Oh Eternal Energy! awaken within us conscious Love, Joy, and Compassion,
conscious Wisdom, Will, Health and Vitality, conscious Realization.
Eternal youth of body and mind abide within us forever.

Prayer for Chi Kung Training

I am an immortal spiritual being, master of this mind body complex.
I direct the energy within me and around me to accumulate
and fill this consciousness with the awareness of Spirit:
Love, Light, Compassion, Truth, Wisdom, Joy, Peace, and Bliss

A Closing Prayer   (from the Bhagavad-Gita)

O Spirit,
I bow to thee in front of me and behind me,
on the left and on the right,
I bow to Thee above and beneath me.
I bow to Thee within and without,
O Lord Omnipresent.

Om Prayer

Oh Great Cosmic Tiger and Dragon;
Creative Omnipotent Power of Om.
With thy song, awaken us into the Unity of Spirit,
As we reverberate and merge with
the Sacred Vibratory Omnipresence of Om.

Prayer used with Wu Tai Hsing "The Form of the Five Elements"

I face the (direction, e.i. east) and behold the day
I am one with Earth and Heaven
Where Fire purifies and Water cleanses.
I am a tree in the wind.
Looking at the world
I gather the best that I see,
I refine it to save what is good
and wash away what is not.
I am one with God.
I embrace the Tiger
and return to the Mountain.

Affirmation of Wu Hsing Chuan "The Form of the Ancient Wisdom of the Five Animals"

The Dragon and Tiger emerge from Spirit.
Together they manifest creation and the souls of humanity.

The Crane and Snake super energize the Lohan and with the knowledge they impart,
the Lohan discovers the Tiger and Dragon at the foundation of his Being
then unites them in the Spiritual Eye.

As the Lohan faces East; Realization Dawns and he becomes the White Panther.
The White Panther merges with Spirit,
chooses and becomes infinite: Light, Love, Compassion, Peace, Wisdom and Joy.

Requirements for Monk Training   **Prayers and Affirmations** - continued

Opening Prayer (for a formal meditation ceremony from Yogacharya Sri John Oliver Black)

Heavenly Father, Divine Mother,
Friend,
Beloved God,
Jesus Christ,
Bhagavan Krishna,
Baba Ji,
Lahiri Mahasaya,
Swami Sri Yukteswar ,
Paramahansa Yogananda
Saints and Sages of all religions,
we bow and recognize the Unity of All.

Free our spiritual paths from all obstacles
and lead us to the shores of eternal Wisdom and Bliss.

May thy Love shine forever
on the sanctuary of our devotion
and we be able to awaken thy Love
in all hearts.

Be thou the only king
reigning on the throne of our consciousness.

Oh Eternal energy,
awaken within us conscious will,
conscious vitality,
conscious health,
conscious realization,
good will to all,
vitality to all,
good health to all,
realization to all.

Eternal youth of body and mind
abide within us forever,
forever,
and forever.

Now with arms upraised to symbolize our upraised consciousness,
let us receive healing for the body, chanting the healing vibrations of Om. Omm.
For the mind. Omm.
And now for the soul. Omm.

Singing Bowl Healing Ritual for Humanity

The Healing Prayer for Humanity
>We are Humanity.
>We are Immortal.
>We are Life.
>We are Love.
>We are Light.
>We are Omnipotent.
>We are Omniscient.
>We are Omnipresent.
>We are Truth.
>We are Wisdom.
>We are Joy.
>We are Peace.
>We are Bliss.
>We are Spirit.

Om Prayer
>Oh Great Cosmic Tiger and Dragon!
>Creative Omnipotent Power of Om.
>With thy song, awaken us and Humanity into the Unity of Spirit,
>As we reverberate and merge with
>the Sacred Vibratory Omnipresence of Om.

Or optionally the Om Prayer from Metaphysical Meditations: Paramahansa Yogananda

As the Frontal Gaze is held and mentally perceiving the self as humanity and Spirit:
 make the bowl sing and chant Omm seven times,
 with each slow inhale, before the chant of each Omm, mentally chant the Humanity Prayer.
The goal is to infuse Humanity with an awareness of Spirit.
This ritual is performed with the focus of this objective in mind.

The Closing Prayer may be used to end the ritual. (An ancient Vedic prayer)
>Oh Spirit!
>I bow to thee in front of me and behind me,
>on the left and on the right,
>I bow to Thee above and beneath me.
>I bow to Thee within and without,
>Oh Lord
>Omnipresent.

Requirements for Monk Training
Healing Ritual - From Yogacharya Sri John Oliver Black

We will now do the healing portion of our ceremony.
Directing our focused attention and using the power of our will, we will send healing energy to where ever we determine it needed.
To do this we are taught to visualize a person or persons or the entire planet within the frontal gaze, surrounded and permeated by God's white healing light.
Do this now holding the focused visualization, and repeat after me:

> Oh! Great Spirit,
> Thou art omnipresent,
> Thou art in all thy children,
> Manifest Thy healing presence
> in their bodies.

> Oh! Great Spirit,
> Thou art omnipresent,
> Thou art in all thy children,
> Manifest Thy healing presence
> in their minds.

> Oh! Great Spirit,
> Thou art omnipresent,
> Thou art in all thy children,
> Manifest Thy healing presence
> in their souls.

Collect energy rubbing the hands together as the prayers are recited,
as each oh the three end, raise the arms overhead releasing the energy and chant OMM, and with the singing of the bowl if it is used.

The Closing Prayer may be used to end the ritual.

Requirements for Monk Training

Lunar Spiritual Eye Energization Ritual

This ritual is performed on the evening of a full moon (or the evening before or the evening after) out side in the presence of the moon, in a place where you will not be distracted.

Create and energize a sacred space.
Pray with the Chi Kung Prayer.
Perform the Staff Ritual to purify and energize the sacred space.
- Perform the formal staff opening with the staff and bow.
- Holding the staff on one end with both hands, repeatedly draw a small clockwise circle above the head while chanting Ommm.
- Continuing the chant and allow the circle to enlarge encompassing the area that will be used for the ritual.
- Finish the Ritual to Energize the Sacred Space with the formal staff close and the bow.

Pray with an opening prayer.

Optionally, energize with the performance of a form, such as: *Wu Tai Hsing, San Zan,* a staff form.

Pray with the Omm prayer.
Perform the last movement of San Zan (breath and the energization visualizations):
1) eighteen times staring into the full moon,
2) as the breath is inhaled add the visualization of drawing the Lunar energy and the rays of light from the moon into your eyes, and directing it to the Upper Dan Tien (Spiritual Eye) at the same, time draw this energy in through the palms of the hands (the Labor Palace) and the mouth with the breath, directing it again to the Upper Dan Tien

On the exhale close the eyes:
1) (instead of dropping the hands) perform the namaskara mudra at the Third Eye
2) and while staring into the light of the Third Eye, chant Omm.

Repeat with each of the eighteen breaths.

Close the sacred space with the <u>Staff Ritual to Energize the Sacred Space</u> by reversing the circle, starting with the large circle and shrinking it to the small circle.

The Closing Prayer may be used to end the ceremony.

Solar Spiritual Eye Energization Ritual

The Lunar Spiritual Eye energization Ritual can be used with the sun as the object for the source of energization. The same steps that are used in the Lunar Ritual are used at dawn and dusk with the sun, as the sun rises and or sets.

Requirements for Monk Training   **Chakra Energization Ritual**   6 - 11

Preparatory Informal Stretching
1) cat, cow   2) shoulder roll   3) neck stretch   4) head to knee   5) rocking chair   6) rocking bow

Posture Instruction
   Hold frontal gaze - performed in each posture
   Series of three posture performances - to stimulate the: body, mind and soul
   Five phases of pose performance
       1) mentally attune   2) sweeping into   3) motionless   4) sweeping out   5) savasana
   alternate forward bend and backward bend; forward bend first, end with backward bend

Formal Energization Routine with Chakra Affirmations and Mantra
1) used to prepare for more efficient energy transportation and raise energy levels in the chakras.
2) forward spinal bend opens centers
3) backward spinal bend moves energy to higher centers
4) performed with Frontal Gaze and mental focus
5) optionally, with affirmation and/or mantra, start with the base chakra first
During phase 3, motionlessness: visualize the chakra with its color, and mentally or audibly recite affirmation, then double exhale and fill the chakra with energy from the inhale, mentally or audibly chanting the mantra 12 times with the beat of the heart, 12 more times with the breath held and 12 more times with the exhale. Then move to the next chakra.

Muladhara Chakra; color: yellow,   mantra: lam
asana: posterior stretch (legs spread), butterfly
I exist in infinite Joy as an entity of Spirit. I prosper in the abundance of Spirit
Swadhishthana Chakra; color: white,   mantra: vam
asana: prone spinal twist, left and right
I exist as infinite Peace in the awareness of Spirit.
           In Bliss I experience the infinite manifestations of Spirit.
Manipura Chakra; color: red,   mantra: ram   asana: bridge, fish
I exist as the omnipotent energy of Spirit. I express compassionate vitality.
Anahata Chakra; color: green-blue,   mantra: yam
asana: seated spinal twist, left and right
I exist as omnipresent Divine Love. With unselfishness and Joy, I serve humanity.
Vishuddha Chakra; color: sea-blue,   mantra: ham
asana: plow, shoulder stand
I exist as Omniscient Wisdom, incarnated as a Bodhisattva
Ajna Chakra, Chandra Chakra; color: snow-white, Spiritual Eye,   mantra: Om
asana: cobra, camel,
I exist as Omnipresent Awareness. Divine Unity is flowing through me.
Sahasrara Chakra; Thousand Petalled-Lotus, brilliant colorless light,   mantra: bam
asana: savasana, or any meditative posture
I exist as the omnipresent brilliance of the spiritual Light.
           I am Spirit. I am Infinite Light, Love, Wisdom, Joy.

Special Event

International Day of Peace Vigil

September 21

Several years ago, the United Nations adopted a resolution designating September 21 of each year as the International Day of Peace with the intention of having the entire world observe a full day of global cease fire and nonviolence. The International Day of Peace Vigil is held on September 21 to use the power of prayer and other spiritual practices in promoting the experience of Peace and preventing violent conflict.

Many religious and spiritual organizations have committed their support. Recently the world Council of Churches invited 550 million people through their member churches to participate in this Vigil. In Sri Lanka, the Sarvodaya Movement expects 200,000 people together in their capital city for a Peace Meditation. Spiritual observances from all religions, groups and individuals worldwide cooperating together will help to unite humanity in the most common cause shared by all - World Peace.

We invite you to send out prayers and meditation for Peace, healing and harmony for all. Every single minute spent in prayer and meditation counts, especially when multiplied by the millions of people throughout the world cooperating in this way! We hope you will plan to share with millions of people in this observance for Peace for humanity and all life on September 21.

Bodhidharma

What you call a temple we call a sangharama, a place of purity. But whoever denies entry to the three klesas and keeps the gates of his senses pure, his body and mind still, inside and outside clean, builds a temple.

Requirements for Monk Training   Days of Commemoration

Days of Commemoration that have been used for ritual purposes.

Spirit and all its aspects, which manifests creation, is at its core and permeates it, are acknowledged. These days are times of energization, self examination, purification, reassessment of perceptions and goals.

These days are usually observed with added discipline such as: meditation, consciousness energization exercises, and fasting.

The Celtic days are included because they are paleolithic, universal and influence all of humanity.

February 2   Imbolc - Celtic
   Marks the first stirrings of spring; a time of magic.

March 1   Holi - Hindu, celebrates the advent of spring

About March 21, at the spring equinox   Ostara - Celtic,
   This is a Fire festival celebrating the resurgence of Earth fertility.

Good Friday and Easter   Mahasamadhi and Resurrection of Jesus

April 9   Chang San Feng - Commemoration Day   Born April 9, 1247   no transition date
   Marks the birth and enlightenment of Chang San Feng.

April 30 or May 1   Beltane - Celtic
   Celebrates the symbolic union of the God and the Goddess; the manifestation of creation.

June 1   Bodhidharma - Commemoration Day   Born 440 A.D.   no transition date
   Marks the birth and enlightenment of Bodhidharma.

May 10   Buddha Purnima
   Hindu - Marks the birth, enlightenment and mahasamadhi of Buddha

About June 21, at the summer solstice   Litha - Celtic
   Marks the point of the year when the Sun is symbolically at the height of its powers.

July 25   Mahavatar Babaji - Commemoration Day   Born November 30, 203   no transition date
   Marks the birth and enlightenment of Babaji

July 27   Nag Panchami   Hindu   Snake Day
   Commemoration of the bestowal of the Cobra Breath to humanity by Babaji

Requirements for Monk Training   **Days of Commemoration** (Continued)

Days of Commemoration that have been used for ritual purposes.

August 1   Lughnasadh - Celtic
   Marks the first harvest and a symbolic ebbing of the Sun's energies.

August 14   Janmashtami   Hindu - Birth of Krishna

September 1   Shri Yogacharya John Oliver Black - Commemoration Day
   Marks the birth, enlightenment and mahasamadhi of Shri Yogacharya John Oliver Black
   Birth September 1, 1893   Mahasamadhi   September 16, 1989

About September 21, the autumnal equinox   Mabon - Celtic
   Marks the second harvest, a time for thanks-giving and reflection.

October 26   Surya Shashti - Hindu   Commemorates the Sun, usually near bodies of water.
   The Solar Spiritual Eye Energization Ritual is usually performed. (Page 6 - 10)
   (Note - Celtic: the Sun can be commemorated daily)

October 31 or November 1   Samhain - Celtic   Sow-in - Irish
   The festival used to gather up energies before the depths of winter.

About December 21, the winter solstice (the days begin to last longer again)   Yule - Celtic
   Marks the rebirth of the Sun, symbolically from the Divine Mother.
   This is a time of Joy and celebration, energization and renewal.

December 25   Birth of Jesus

On the occasion of the each full Moon   Esbat – Celtic   Chandra Shashti – Hindu
   This is a celebration of the Divine Mother and the Heavenly Father (which is reflected in
   the Divine Mother), just as the Sun is reflected in the Moon.
   The Lunar Spiritual Eye Energization Ritual is usually performed. (Page 6 - 10)
   This is a time of energization and renewal.

Mudra

Mudra are movements and postures of the body, an appendage or hand that can call our attention to a spiritual concept or aspect of Spirit. Mudra are imbued with and have energy of their own, because they have been practice by thousands of people for centuries; even millennia. They are used by monks in their spiritual exercises of prayer, ritual, ritual movement, ceremony, concentration and meditation. They are also used to teach spiritual concepts to monks.

High levels of psychic energy, will and mental focus are required for efficient meditation. Mudra performance during meditation can assist in raising energy levels and mental focus.

Considerably more energy and mental application are required to communicate audibly using mantra than mudra during meditation. Physical communication with mudra can be more energy efficient and less disturbing to the consciousness than audible communication. This can make mudra use more efficient than mantra or affirmations.

The energy and the concept of a mudra can be experienced in the performance of the mudra. The Form of the Five Elements (Wu Tai Hsing) is a mudra of movement, that can move the consciousness into an awareness of being part of nature and Spirit. The inclusion of mudra in the practice of forms, will make the forms practice a ritual of spiritual insight, affirmation and a recommitment to the inner work.

The use of mudra begins with knowledge of the meaning of each mudra practiced.

To obtain efficient results from mudra training within the performance of forms, these five criteria must be met.

1) The forms must be performed in a state of wu hsin.
2) The practitioner must have intellectual knowledge of the meaning of the mudra practiced
3) The personality must have matured enough to realize the truth of the meaning of the mudra
4) The results are enhanced with the silent recitation of the name of the mudra as it is performed
5) The forms practice must have a disciplined schedule, a minimum of three or four days a week.
  This repetition of practice will have greater influence than repeated hypnotic suggestion.

If the physical health requirements are met (nutrition, sleep, hygiene, etc.) vitality levels, mental health and mental acuity will rise.
The realized results will develop and instill spiritual perception.
Stress and suffering will diminish in direct proportion to the development of spiritual perception.
Divine Love, Light, Wisdom and Joy will develop in direct proportion to the development of spiritual perception.

Mudra List

While there are a large number of esoteric mudra, what follows are the most common mudra used within the Shaolin Tradition.

Page

1) Abaya Mudra.....................................6 - 17
2) Varada Mudra....................................6 - 17
3) Dharma Chakra Mudra......................3 - 18
4) Namaste   Anjali Mudra....................6 - 18
5) Nataraja Mudra.................................6 - 19
6) Dhyani Mudra...................................6 - 19
7) Buddha Shramana Mudra..................6 - 20
8) Bhumisparsha Mudra........................6 - 20
9) Vajrapradama Mudra.........................6 - 20
10) Dharma-megha Mudra.....................6 - 21
11) Bhujang Mudra................................6 - 22
12) The Immortal Man Points the Way...6 - 22
13) He Mudra..6 - 23
14) Om Mudra......................................6 - 23
15) Dhrithi Mudra..................................6 - 23
16) Ishvara Mudra.................................6 - 24
17) The Heaven and Earth Mudra..........6 - 24
18) Pai She Shuochu Xin.......................6 - 24

The Mudra of the Five Elements:
19) Wood...6 - 25
20) Fire..6 - 25
21) Earth..6 - 25
22) Metal...6 - 25
23) Water...6 - 25
24) Ether / Spirit...................................6 - 25

Mudra Combinations
25) San Sao...6 - 26
26) San Sao Er.....................................6 - 26
27) Er Sao..6 - 26
28) San Sao to the Heavens.................6 - 26
29) The Five Steps................................6 - 26
30) Pai He Liang Chi.............................6 - 26
List of Mudra within the Forms..............6 - 27

Requirements for Monk Training Mudra: Symbolism and Use - Continued 6 - 17

1) Abaya Mudra - Mudra of Peace

Both hands or one hand are held flat (fingers and palm) and vertical with the thumbs tucked, in front of the shoulder or center in front of the throat.

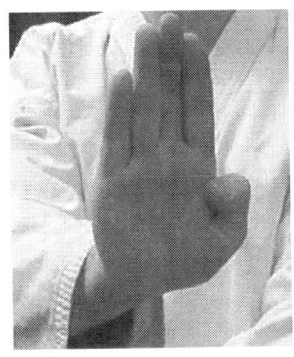

This mudra is a request for divine assistance in the incorporation of Peace, and Fearlessness (and the aspects of Spirit) into ones personality. This concept of fearlessness is aimed at the courage required to face and defeat the klesic demons of self centeredness, ignorance, and fear. This victory is a prerequisite for complete spiritual realization.

With the defeat of the inner demons one becomes a being on Infinite Peace. The mudra becomes a sign of non-aggression, protection, blessing, reassurance and compassion for others.

The personality must be purified to completely experience Spirit.

The amount of spiritual realization one attains is directly proportional to how well the aspects of Spirit are integrated into the personality.

Some aspects of Spirit include: Divine Love, Light, Compassion, Truth, Wisdom, Joy, Peace, Unity, Bliss.

Mudra affirmation:
   I am an immortal spiritual being of Infinite Peace and fearlessness.
   Fearless, I will face and defeat the demons within.

2) Varada Mudra - The mudra of the Five Perfections

One hand or both are held flat (fingers and palm) and vertical, fingers pointing down, with the thumbs tucked, at the hip or center out in front of the navel.

This mudra is a request for divine assistance in the incorporation of the Five Perfections into the personality. It symbolizes the bestowal of the Five Perfections; the supreme accomplishment. The Five Perfections is a template used in the process of Self Examination\Personality Purification for the development of spiritual realization.

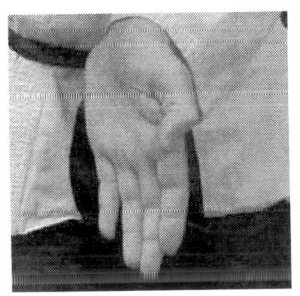

1) Perfect Compassion develops Perfect Charity
2) Perfect Love develops Perfect Morality
3) Perfect Determination develops Perfect Patience
4) Perfect Discipline develops Perfect Effort
5) Perfect Concentration/Meditation develops Enlightenment

The delusion of pride and separateness is transformed into Compassion, equality and the experience of Unity.

Mudra affirmation:
   I am an immortal spiritual being,
         transformed by the Five Perfections,
               I am devoted to the salvation of humanity.

6 - 18   **Requirements for Monk Training   Mudra: Symbolism and Use - Continued**

3) Dharma Chakra Mudra (the Turning of the Wheel of Cosmic Law, also, the Setting into Motion the Wheel of the Teaching of the Dharma)

This mudra is a request for divine assistance in the process of personality purification and the dissolution of the karmic debt. This mudra sets into motion the turning of the wheel of dharmic teaching and the exposure of karmic influences. It will bring into your life situations and circumstances that will expose the limitations within your personality that must be eliminated. The delusion of ignorance is transformed, by the integration of wisdom of the imagined self, into Wisdom of the Great Self.

The first version of the Dharma Chakra Mudra, is the simultaneous performance of three mudra: 1) the circle formed by the rotation of the 2) Abaya and 3)Varada Mudra. This version is also known as the San Sao Mudra .

A variation of this mudra is performed by touching the tips of the index finger and thumbs of both hands (as in the Om Mudra), slightly extending the three remaining fingers of each hand and placing the hands in front of the heart, with the left palm slightly inward and the right palm slightly outward. The three slightly extended fingers of the left hand represent the Triratna (the Buddha, the Dharma, and the Sangha). The three slightly extended fingers of the right hand represent the "hearers" of the teachings, solitary realizers' and the teachings. This version is sometimes called The Reach into the Dark.

Mudra affirmation:
	I am totally committed to the process of complete personality purification and request divine assistance in the accomplishment of this process.

	In perfect Peace I walk the path of the Five Perfections.

4) Namaste Mudra or **Anjali Mudra** - The Prayer Mudra, The Mudra of Humility

Palms of the hands placed together, fingers pointing up and thumbs tucked in front of the heart; often performed with a bow.

This is the mudra of respect and humility. It is used as a greeting and for prayer. The delusion of separateness transforms into the awareness of Spiritual Unity. This mudra is an acknowledgment of the microcosmic self, existing as a part of the Great Self (Spirit).

Mudra affirmation:
		I behold the infinite eternal Life of Love and Compassion
			that exists within you, within me,
				and exists within all of creation and beyond.

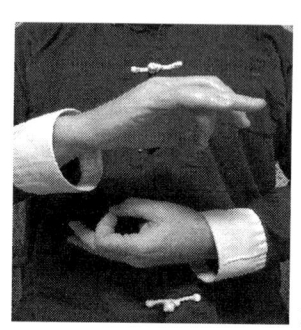

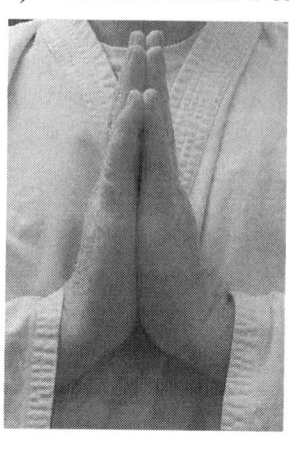

Requirements for Monk Training **Mudra: Symbolism and Use** - Continued   6 - 19

5) Nataraja Mudra

Both hands hold the Buddha Shramana Mudra. The arms are moved with speed and placed in positions that simulate the multiple arms of Shiva in the aspect of the Nataraja (the cosmic dancer). Shiva, in the Nataraja aspect, is responsible for all change within creation. Change is the catalyst of constructive experience.

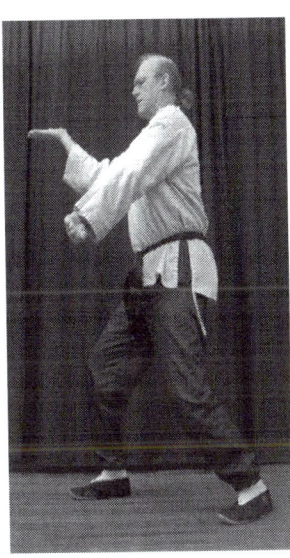

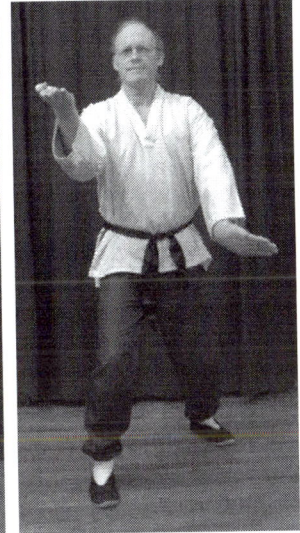

The multiple arms represent Spirit and in the aspects of immortality, omnipotence, omniscience, omnipresence. When the mudra is performed it is calling the attention to the awareness of Spirit which is at the core of our own being.

Mudra affirmation:
   I realize at the core of my being I am Spirit, encompassing all of its aspects: immortality, omnipotence, omniscience, omnipresence, Love, Light, Compassion, Truth, Wisdom, Joy, Peace, Bliss.

6) Dhyani - Meditation Mudra

The hands are placed in the lap, palms up, one hand on top of the other, thumbs raised and touching. The thumbs raised and touching represents the spiritual fire that consumes all impurities.

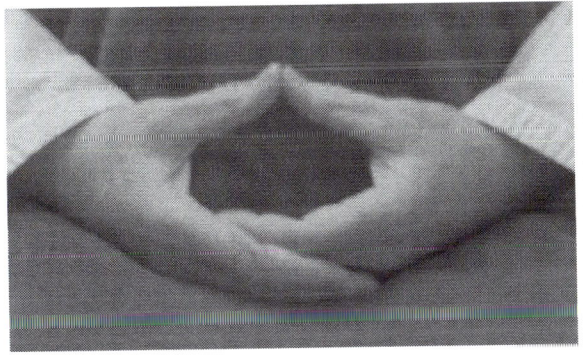

The delusion of attachment transforms to Wisdom of discernment.
This mudra will effect mental balance in meditation. It will assist in sense withdrawal and tranquility.
This mudra assists in the accomplishment of Chitta-Vritti-Nirodha; mastery of the mind. Mental mastery is prerequisite to true meditation.

Mudra affirmation: My being rests in the Supreme Awareness.

7) Buddha Shramana Mudra

The flat hand, fingers and tucked thumb are placed palm up and horizontal, usually shoulder high in front of and just outside of the shoulder.

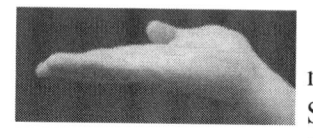

This mudra represents: the realization of existing in a state without misery, stepping out of the worldly paradigm into the awareness of the Spiritual reality and a commitment to not participate in the *competition* for power, security and survival that is predominate in the cultures and social norms of the world. This is the affirmation of the renunciant.

Mudra affirmation:
   I am an immortal spiritual being, while I live in this world, I will not be part of it.

8) Bhumisparsha Mudra

The flat hand, fingers and tucked thumb are placed palm down and horizontal, usually out in front of the navel or high in front of and just outside of the shoulder or at times, flat on the floor.

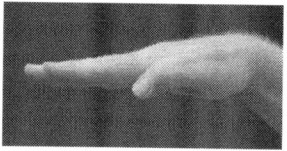

This is a gesture of "touching the Earth" that the Buddha performed when he made the Divine Mother aware of his initial experience of God Realization. It has come to indicate that what has been said is Truth; and like Truth, is unchangeable. This is very similar to what the word Amen has come to mean in the Christian Tradition.

Mudra affirmation: As the Lord is my witness, this is Truth.

9) Vajrapradama Mudra

The flat hands, fingers and tucked thumb are held flat and diagonally placed with the fingers crossing in front of the navel center. The navel center, the Lower Tan Tien, is the source of energy within our being.

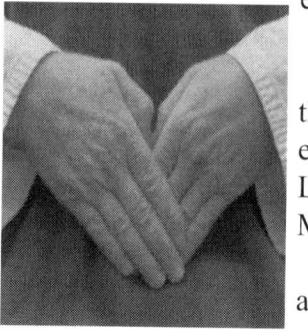

Vajra means lightening bolt and is referring to the super brilliance of the Spiritual Light. The sustained experience of this light will bring enlightenment; an awareness of Spirit in all its aspects. An aspect of Light that our attention is attracted to is Wisdom. The Vajrapradama Mudra calls our attention to these aspects of Spirit within ourselves.

It is performed at the beginning and end of some forms. Examples are the Kushanku and Naihanchin kata.

This mudra has the same meaning as that of the closed fists; absolute resolve, unshakable confidence.

Mudra affirmation: The Light of Spiritual Wisdom permeates this being.

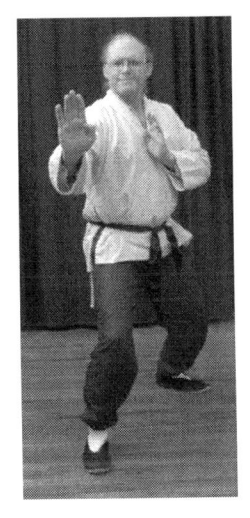

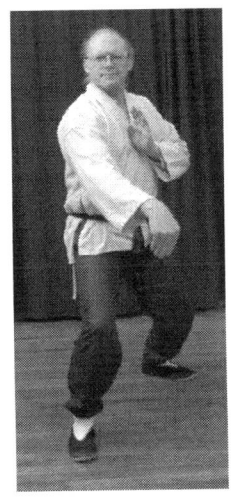

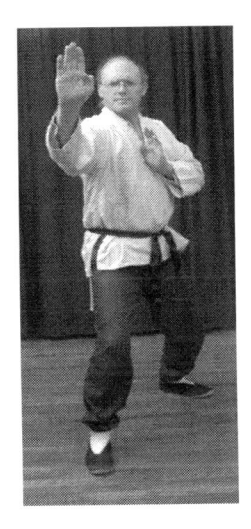

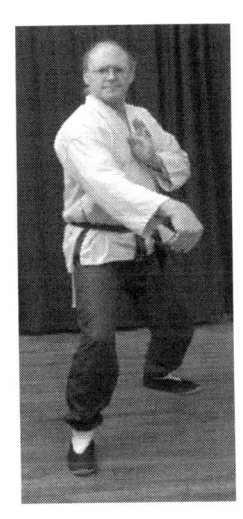

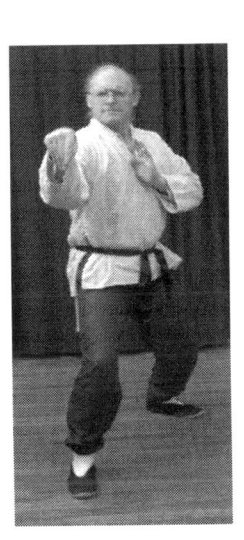

Requirements for Monk Training **Mudra: Symbolism and Use** - Continued   6 - 21

10) Dharma-Megha Mudra

One arm draws a large oval in front of the torso as the wrist bends the open hand, up and down; as in "paint the fence". Drawing this large oval symbolizes the dissolution of the ones attachments and karmic debt. The movement is completed with the Bujang Mudra. The bujang Mudra symbolizes the Shaolin spiritual training methods of the Snake and the Cobra Breath technique. Ending the Dharma-Megha Mudra with the Bujang Mudra is an affirmation that the Shaolin Tradition and its spiritual training is what one is using to accomplish the dissolution of one's attachments and karmic debt.

Picture 1   The movement starts as the right hand comes down on the right side of the torso with the fingers pointing up and dropping to the level of the waist.
Picture 2   The hand travels to the left side of the torso and rises with the fingers pointing down.
Picture 3   The hand travels to the right side again and drops.
Picture 4   The hand travels to the left side then rises diagonally to the point in front of the heart.
Picture 5   The hand finishes the oval in front of the shoulder with the Bujang Mudra.

The delusion of bondage and limitation is burned in the fire of purification and all that is left is realization of the Supreme Reality. This is the mudra of the dissolution of the karmic debt and all attachment. With the dissolution of the karmic debt and attachment, the causes of bondage and limitation are removed. This is the last level of samadhi before total realization occurs. The soul spreads its wings of Wisdom as it is released from maya and rises into the radiant brilliance of Spirit and awareness of all its aspects.

Mudra affirmation:
    I am Divine Spirit,
        I am one with the Brilliant Omnipresent Spiritual Light
            of Infinite Love, Wisdom and Bliss.

11) Bhujang Mudra — Cobra Snake Mudra

The thumb touches the index and middle finger, and the wrist is bent forward palm down. The mudra is usually placed in front of the heart or center in front of the throat.

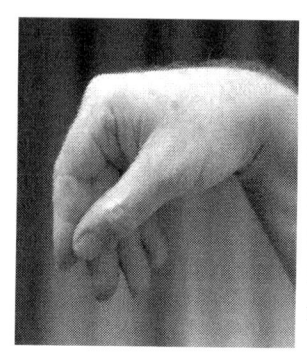

This mudra refers to the commitment-vow to use the Shaolin Tradition (which includes the Cobra Breath) to accomplish spiritual realization. The cobra snake represents the spinal cord, medulla, and brain (because of the similarity in appearance and the use of this path in the Cobra Breath chi kung). These are the principle organs used in the energization of consciousness. The energization of consciousness is required to expand the awareness sufficiently to experience spiritual realization.

This mudra usually ends the performance of the Dharma-Megha Mudra. When these mudra are performed together, the monk is stating the goal of his or her life; the purification of the consciousness and with the performance of the Bhujang Mudra, the method of obtaining spiritual illumination is reaffirmed.

Mudra affirmation: I am a Shaolin Bodhisattva Monk,
          using the methods of the Shaolin Tradition
                 to obtain complete God Realization.

12) The Immortal Man Points the Way

The index and middle fingers are extended straight and point. The little and ring fingers curl toward the palm. The thumb is place on top of the nails of these fingers and holds them in place.

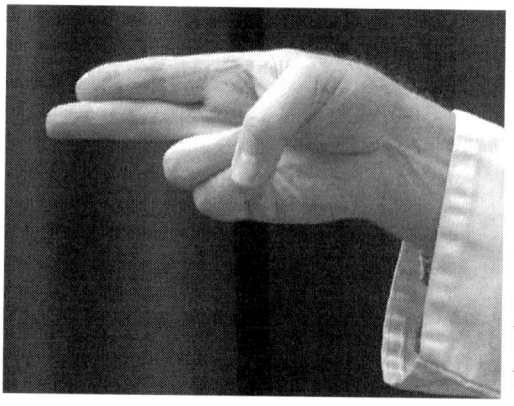

Ultimately Spirit/God is the guru. At the core of our being we are Spirit/Reality, Truth. The Immortal Man is the guru within (Truth). (Truth, with a capital T, is an aspect of Spirit). The Truth will point the way whether you ignore it or not. When Truth is ignored it is ignorance. The klesa of ignorance is the root cause of all stress and suffering. When Truth is fully experienced, all stress and suffering will end and all the aspects of Spirit will blossom in the awareness. The Immortal Man Points the Way.

Mudra affirmation: The Immortal Man points the Way.

13) He Mudra - The Crane Mudra

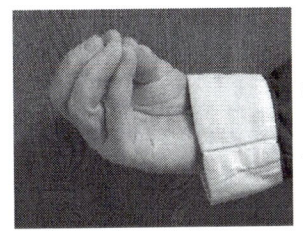

The wrist bends forward and the tip of the thumb and the tips of all four fingers are brought together and touch at the same time.

The Crane represents Wisdom and the knowledge of the synergy of the physical body, mind and soul awareness, while the consciousness is incarnated on Earth. The development of any one of these aspects of the self will increase the potential for the development of the other two. The strength and vitality of the physical body dramatically enhances the ability of incarnate beings to interact with the environment of the world. Not only does it enhance the Joy of the experience, but also enhances mental function. Enhanced mental function is usually prerequisite for the development of spiritual realization. So the Wisdom of the Crane encompasses the spiritual methods and techniques of the physical training within the Shaolin Tradition. The Wisdom of the Crane, is used as preparation for the spiritual training and the spiritual experience.

Mudra affirmation: As a Shaolin Bodhisattva Warrior, I dedicate my life to the elimination of the suffering of all beings.

14) Om Mudra \ Buddha Mudra \ Ghana Mudra

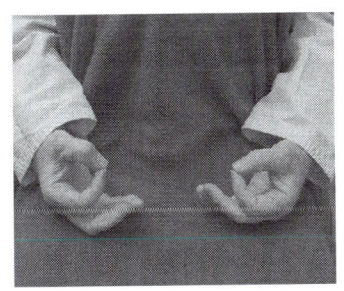

The tip of the thumb touches the tip of the index finger. The thumb (represents God) and the index finger (represents the personality) with the circle formed by the two, they merge into One.

Ghana Mudra (Wisdom) A variation is the index finger placed on the center of pad of the thumb.

The Buddha Mudra is performed by assuming the Om Mudra with both hands, palms up, placed in the lap or on the knees.

It is used during meditation. Also, this mudra can be of assistance when practicing the Om Meditation. This mudra assists the consciousness in the mental mastery required for true meditation. Aggressive thoughts and behaviors transform into Peace and tranquility. The human soul becomes balanced into perfect harmony with Spirit in all its aspects.

Mudra affirmation: I exist in perfect Peace.

15) Dhrithi Mudra - The Closed Fists

The closed fist or fists are a mudra of total commitment, confidence, absolute resolve, emphasizing a statement of fact with a recognition of Self Divinity within Unity

Mudra affirmation: As a Being of Spirit, I will make this happen.

Requirements for Monk Training   **Mudra: Symbolism and Use** - Continued

16) Ishvara Mudra Mudra of Spirit - Ishvara (the Indwelling Reality)

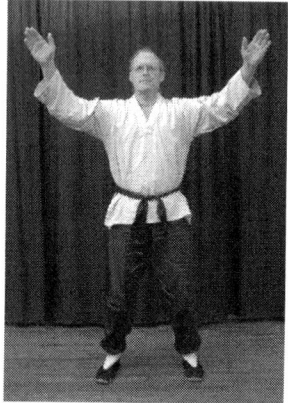

The Ishvara Mudra is a movement, that begins with the hands placed in the Anjali Mudra. The hands rise together above the head, separate and spread apart in a large circle, dropping to low center, the point where the hands are together again, and then rise together to the Anjali Mudra once more. If the feet are apart the left knee is lifted and the left foot steps to the right foot as the circle is drawn. Also the breath is usually inhaled as the circle is drawn (filling the awareness with Spirit).

Ishvara is the sanskrit term for the Great Spirit. As the body rises with the arms spread apart above the head, this mudra represents Rising into Spirit. It calls our attention to the energy and influence of Spirit that permeates the universe and experiencing the aspects of Spirit within our own awareness.

Mudra affirmation: This consciousness returns to the awareness of the Ultimate Reality.

17) Heaven and Earth Mudra *Mudra of Life - Embrace the Tiger and Return to the Mountain*:

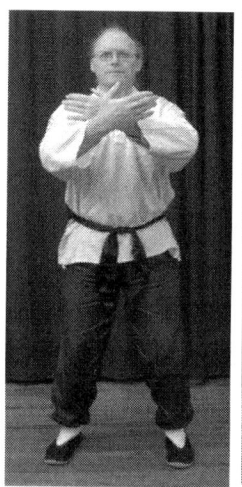

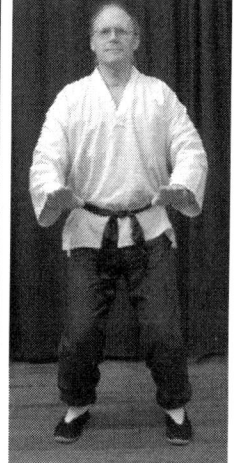

The hands spread out to the sides at waist level, move downward and to the center. Then the wrists cross as the hands rise palms facing toward the chest. The hands then turn over palms down and the elbows straighten (but not completely) as the hands are pushed toward the floor.

In Chinese cosmology the Tiger symbolizes the Divine Mother and all that She represents: Life, Love, Light, Wisdom, Joy, all the aspects of Spirit. To embrace the Tiger, means that we embrace, with enthusiasm and joy, all that she represents and all the experiences and learning that our existence brings. The mountain is gigantic and almost infinite like Spirit and therefore, represents Spirit. At the end of the experience of life on Earth, or the limited self consciousness, we return to life in Spirit and the awareness of Spirit in all its aspects.

Mudra affirmation: I Embrace the Tiger and Return to the Mountain.

18) Pai She Shuochu Xin *The White Snake Speaks Truth*

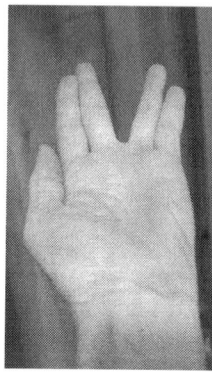

The White Snake refers to the Shaolin spiritual chi kung, spiritual knowledge and Truth. The White Snake also represents the cerebral-spinal pathway. This is the path used in the Shaolin spiritual chi kung to energize the consciousness. The middle fingers spread represents the tongue of the snake. The tongue is used in spiritual chi kung to stimulate the spiritual eye (the upper tan tien) to enhance intuition, spiritual insight and meditation. The White Snake Speaks Truth is referring to the results of the White Snake training. Not only is the White Snake training Truth but it bestows the Great Truth to the trainee.

Requirements for Monk Training   Mudra: Symbolism and Use - Continued   6 - 25

The Five Elements (Wu Xing): **19)** Wood (Mu)   **20)** Fire (Hou)   **21)** Earth (Tu)
22) Metal (Jin)   **23)** Water (Shui)   plus the source of the five   **24)** Ether / Spirit (Shen)
In Chinese cosmology these elements refer not to matter but to elemental energies that interact with each other to produce our material realm. The Creator uses these 5 elements in the process of manifesting creation. Each element is represented with a movement and posture within the form which are mudra. The performance of these mudra can help make us aware of these elemental energies within ourselves and of our relationship to creation.

Wood

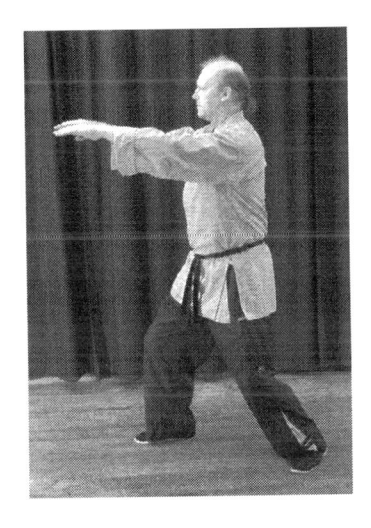

Fire

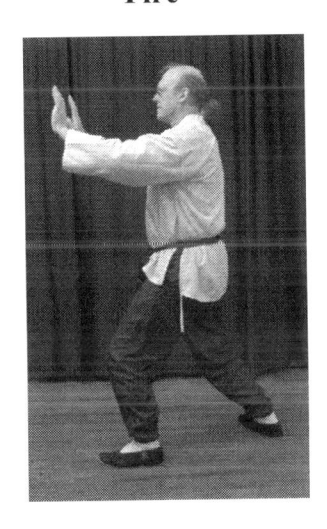

Earth

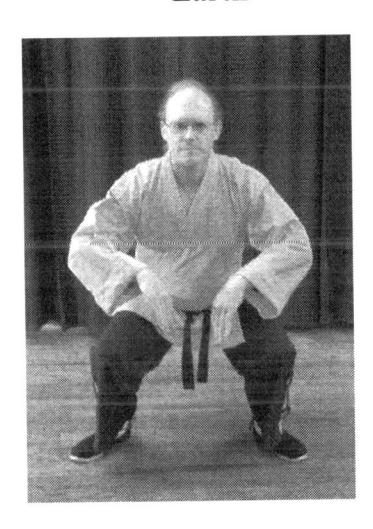

Metal

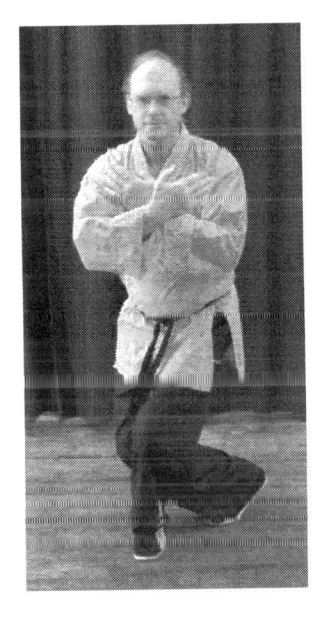

Water

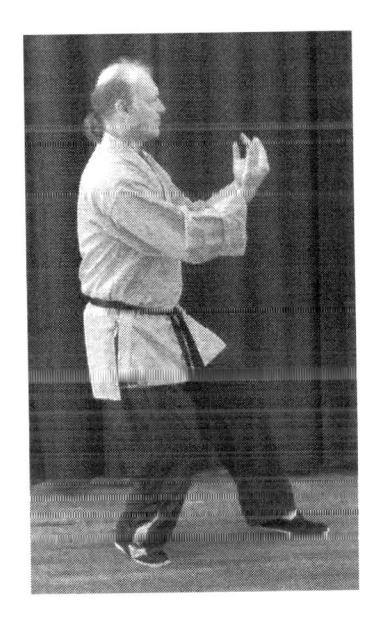

Ether / Spirit

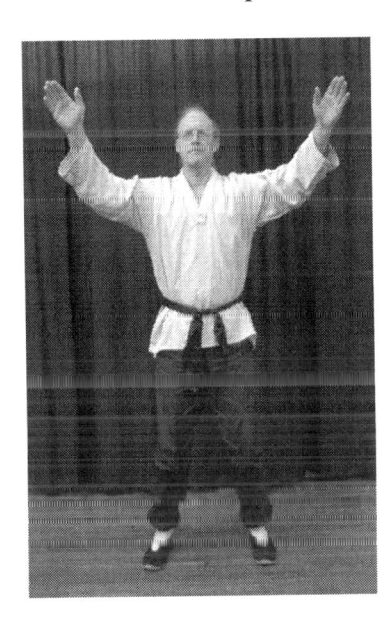

Mudra Combinations

25) San Sao - The Simultaneous performance of 3 Mudra
   This is a version of the Dharma Chakra Mudra. The San Sao Mudra is performed by drawing a circle formed by the rotation of the Abaya Mudra in one hand and Varada Mudra in the other. As the hands rotate, each mudra turns into the other. This is a request for divine assistance in the development of the power of the will, specifically for the process of defeating the klesic demons and in the incorporation of the Five Perfections into ones consciousness.
   San Sao is performed in:
            San Zan Chuan, Sei San Chuan, San Sei Chuan, Wu Shi Si, Bodhisattva Tao.
The mudra affirmation of San Sao is: In Perfect Peace I walk the path of the Five Perfections.

26) San Sao Er - Mudra of the Renunciant
   In the San Sao Er Mudra, the circle formed by the rotation of the Abaya Mudra and Bhumisparsha Mudra. This is a request for divine assistance in the removal of the worldly paradigm from ones consciousness.
   Performed in the hsing: Wu Shi Si, Pai She Chuan

27) Er Sao
   The simultaneous performance of Buddha Shramana and Bhumisparsha.
ER Sao is performed in the hsing: Pai He Chuan, Bodhisattva Tao, San Sei Chuan

28) San Sao to the Heavens
   This version of the San Sao Mudra is performed with a horizontal rotation of the Buddha Shramana in each hand as in the Dharma Chakra Mudra in Pai He Hsing. This is a double request for divine assistance in the removal of the worldly paradigm from ones consciousness.

29) The Five Steps
   The series of five steps taken in many of the forms represent the path of the Five Perfections and the vow-commitment to its use in the development of spiritual awareness.
The Five Steps are performed in the hsing:
San Zan Chuan   San Sei Chuan   Sei San Chuan   Pai She Chuan   Bodhisattva Tao

30) Pai He Liang Chi - The White Crane Spreads Its Wings
   This mudra is a circular rotation and double presentation of the Buddha Shramana and Bumisparsha Mudra, moving through and sometimes finishing with the Crane Stance. This is a request for divine assistance in the removal of the worldly paradigm from ones consciousness.

Requirements for Monk Training   Mudra: Symbolism and Use - Continued

Lists of Mudra within Temple Forms

The Mudra of San Zan Chuan (The Ancient Wisdom of the Three Battles):
Varada Mudra	Bhumis Parsha Mudra	San Sao Mudra
Abaya Mudra	Dharma-Megha Mudra	
Bujang Mudra	Buddha Shramana Mudra	

The Mudra of Wu Hsing Chuan (The Form of the Five Animals):
Anjali
- Dragon — Lung
- Tiger — Hu
- Crane — He
- Snake — She
- Panther — Bao
- Ishvara

Abaya Mudra
Bhumisparsha Mudra
Buddha Shramana Mudra
Pai She Shouchu Xin - The White Snake Speaks Truth

Mudra of Wu Tai Hsing (The Form of the Five Elements)
Anjali   Abaya Mudra   Ishvara Mudra   Bhumisparsha Mudra   Heaven and Earth Mudra

5 Elements (Wu Xing):
1) Fire, Hou   2) Water, Shui   3) Wood, Mu   4) Metal, Jin   5) Earth, Tu

The Mudra of Pai He Chuan (Form of the Ancient Wisdom of the White Crane)
Anjali Mudra	San Sao Mudra	Bhumis Parsha Mudra	Varada Mudra
Abaya Mudra	Pai He Liang Chi	Buddha Shramana Mudra	Dhrithi Mudra

The Mudra of Wu Shi Si:
Buddha Shramana	Dharma Chakra Mudra	Nataraja	He Mudra
Bhumis Parsha	Dharma Mega Mudra	Bhujang	Abaya Mudra

The Mudra of Pai She Chuan (Form of the Ancient Wisdom of the White Snake)
Anjali - Ishvara Mudra	Bujang Mudra	Abaya Mudra
Varada Mudra	Dharma-Megha Mudra	Buddha Shramana Mudra
Heaven and Earth	Nataraja - San Sao II	Bhumis Parsha Mudra

PART VII

MONASTIC INITIATION and MONASTIC REQUIREMENTS
GRADING AND EVALUATION

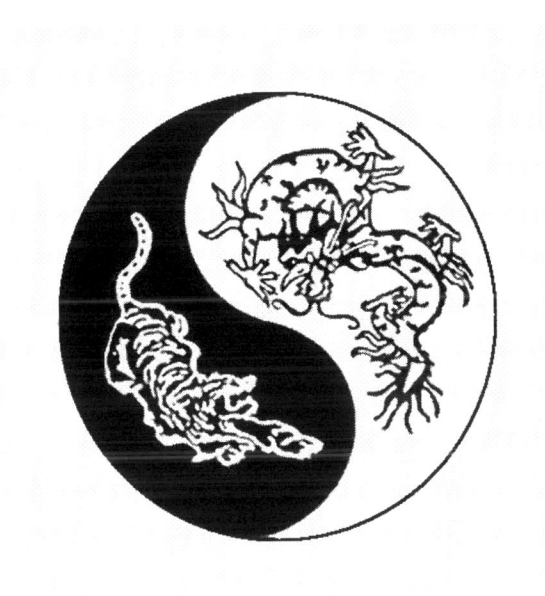

Monastic Requirements   **General Grading Information**

Criteria for the Evaluation of Hsing

General Grading Information

Level requirements are cumulative for each advancement. In addition to the requirements for each advancement, the monk must also be able to meet the requirements of the previous test or tests.

The technique requirements of each advancement must be performed before the judging teacher(s) a sufficient number of times to permit the determination of proficiency.

The criteria for evaluation of technique combinations and forms are the same for every level.

The grading system has been established for four reasons:
1) It is a means of structuring the presentation of the knowledge to be disseminated in a way to make the learning process more efficient.
2) The learning process is broken into blocks that are used as short term goals. Goal setting is used to keep up the sustained effort required to succeed in a timely manner.
3) The grading system can aid students in the selection of learning facilitators.
4) The grading system is used to prepare the student for the more advanced training that requires prerequisite skills and abilities.

Criteria for the Evaluation of Hsing
Each movement must be performed:

- in the required sequence
- with the required focus of the eyes, body, mind and breath
- with the required stance and posture
- with the required coordination and placement of eyes, hands and feet
- at the angle of the required movement direction
- with the required speed, balance and fluidity
- each Hsing will be performed at least twice
    1) Once with the count of the instructor
    2) And once without the count of the instructor

"Judge not that ye be not judged. For with what judgement ye judge, ye shall be judged; and with what measure ye mete, it shall be measured to you again."
                                        - Jesus   Matthew 7: 1-2

Criteria for Evaluation of Written Assignments

An <u>essay</u> will require at least two full pages of content.

A <u>research paper</u> will require at least ten full pages of content.

Aspects of writing that will be evaluated are:

- topic coverage
- unnecessary turn offs
- identifiable structure - example
    - A. introductory paragraph with guiding sentence
    - B. body paragraphs which discuss guiding sentence
    - C. conclusion paragraph that summarizes
- writing style (do the ideas blend?)
- cover page
- outline page
- footnotes
- bibliography page
- word spelling
- use of punctuation
- use of capitalization
- word usage
- phrase construction (syntax)
- sentence structure
- paragraph structure

Tao Te Ching
Lao Tzu
Chapter 34

Supreme is the Tao! All pervasive; it is on the left hand and on the right.
All things depend on it for life, and it denies none.
Its purposes accomplished, it claims no credit.
It clothes and fosters all things, but claims no lordship.
Ever desireless, it may be named "The Indivisible."
All things revert to it, but it claims no lordship.
      It may be named "The Supreme."
Because to the end the sage does not seek supremacy;
      he is able to accomplish great things.

Monastic Requirements   **Requirements for Student Monk**

I. General
- A. Regular class attendance (at least twice a week)
- B. Age - must be at least Fourteen years old
- C. Vow (page 6-3)

II. Crane Requirements
- A. Forms
  1. San Zan (performed at least once a day with the 5 Perfections Affirmations)
- B. Chi Kung - Explain and demonstrate:
  1. The Abdominal Breath
  2. Energization Tension Rotation Exercise (page 4 - 18)
  3. Crane Breath (practice one round of 18 breaths before each meditation)

III. Snake Requirements
- A. Must know the Opening Prayer
- B. Must know the Energization Prayer
- C. Must meditate at least two times each day (best times are at dawn, dusk, noon, midnight)
- D. Vow practice, as one rises and retires.
- E. Know and practice the Omm Mantra Meditation after Crane Breath practice

IV. Academic
- A. Understand and Explain the Goals and Methods of the Shaolin Tradition
- B. Understand and Explain the Energization of Consciousness Concept
- C. Understand and Explain the Purification of Consciousness Concept
- D. Be able to define the Spirit of Ken Do
- E. Be able to explain the reason for the Jyu Gong (bow) and when it should be performed.
- F. Show the ability to conduct the class opening and closing ceremonies and define the meaning of the words used.
- G. Be able to count to ten in Chinese.
- H. Own and read the Monk Manual
- I. Read two books and submit a written paragraph on each of the 25 most important points in each book (Books are assigned by the director)

V. Character
- A. Integrity
- B. Has made self development an ultimate concern
- C. Has accepted a self disciplined life
- D. Has accepted responsibility for all of ones behaviors and all of ones circumstances.
- E. Has established a daily habit of consciousness energization, meditation and prayer

VI. Leadership
- A. Accept responsibility for the facilitation of holistic growth of self and all others
- B. Show competency in directing discipline in the Tao Chang

Student Monk: Testing Information
The Spirit of Ken Do and the Training Uniform (Do Gi)

The training uniform is a traditional symbol of the spirit of Ken Do. This spirit is an attitude and a code of conduct that is basically taught by all the major religions and philosophies of the world. Fundamentally the principles of the spirit of Ken Do are:

- that we should never do wrong or return a wrong, in thought or deed,

- that we are responsible, to the best of our abilities, to help all people and our selves, toward a positive mental, physical and spiritual development,

- and that we are responsible for our own actions; we do not do anything we are told to do unless we know from within ourselves that it is proper.

The mental strength derived from the dedicated practice of kung fu combined with the mental and spiritual assimilation of the spirit of Ken Do leads the seeker to the goal of perfection. The pursuit of perfection has been illustrated by the washing away of imperfect thoughts and deeds; as in the Christian baptism where sins are washed away with clean water. Water, being clear and transparent has been associated with the color white, which is clear and free of the impurities of other colors.

In a sense you are wearing a baptism when you wear a training uniform. It is a visible symbol of the commitment you have made to yourself to comply with the spirit of Ken Do. It shows all who see it that you have the best interests of everyone at heart.

The Tradition of the Bow with Namaste

The bow is a simple ritual that also signifies your compliance to the spirit of Ken Do. This ritual is performed as we enter and leave the Tao Chang as an acknowledgment of respect for the place and the seriousness of the reasons we are there. It is performed as we begin practice with any individual or group to show that we have their best interests at heart, that we will use the care and control to keep any injuries from happening and that we will do our best to make the practice as productive as possible. The bow is also performed during the class openings and closings, and optionally to each other or anyone, anytime, or anywhere.

Monastic Requirements   **Student Monk: Testing Information** (continued)

Class Opening and Closing Ceremonies

Chinese	English
Pai duei	line up
Hsiu Hsing	Prepare for self purification training (stand at attention)
Zhouxia	formal seated, *vajrasan* (knees and insteps on floor. Seated on heels)
Kwan Kung	Ceremonial Bow (to perceive the Infinite)
Qidao	Opening Prayer (required when a monk opens class)
He Huxi	Crane Breath
Chan na	Meditation
Ting zhi	stop (end meditation)
Xiang sifu jyu gong	Bow to tradition
Kai shi	begin (for opening ceremony)
Jai san	disperse (for closing ceremony)

Numbers	Chinese
one	yi
two	er
three	san
four	si
five	wu
six	liu
seven	qu
eight	ba
nine	jiu
ten	shi

Opening Prayer

Oh Divine Ultimate All! Of Infinite Light, Love, Wisdom, and Joy!,
In dweller within the fabric of all of Creation and Beyond,
unto you do we turn our consciousness.

Teach us to completely Love All,
To perceive ourselves in All,
To fully experience our Divine Unity and Immortality.

Teach us detachment from all worldliness.
Bring us the Wisdom that will deliver us from delusion,
Instill within us perfectly positive thought, removing all negativity and fear.
Experiencing self mastery and complete Self Realization,
as Infinite Light, Love, Wisdom, Joy, The Divine Ultimate All.

7 - 6   Monastic Requirements   Reading Requirements for Student Monk

Student Monk: Academic Reading Requirements Description

Read Two Books: director assigned books

As each book is read, the testee will take notes on the most important points each book makes. The notes on the most important points made in each chapter will be submitted. Also, when the testee has finished reading each book, the 25 most important points the book makes will be selected. A paragraph explaining each of the 25 most important points will be submitted (25 paragraphs, one on each point), on each of the two books. In addition the testee **may** submit 25, four answer, multiple choice questions concerning each of the most important points, on each book. The testee will have the option of orally presenting the tests to a class.

Autobiography of a Yogi   Paramahansa Yogananda   ISBN 1-56589-108-2
The Bodhisattva Warriors   Shifu Nagaboshi Tomio   ISBN 0-87728-785-6

'The disciple is not above his master: but every one that is perfect shall be as his master."
- Jesus   Luke 6:40

Jesus on the Influence of Law and Rules

"Woe unto you, lawyers! For you have taken away the key of knowledge: Ye entered not in yourselves, and them that were entering in ye hindered."   - Jesus   Luke 11: 52

The *key of knowledge* is *entering into your self.*
Here the use of the word *knowledge* includes Wisdom and spiritual perception.

Monastic Requirements   **Requirements for Disciple Monk**

I. General
  A. At least six months as a Student Monk,
  with regular class attendance (at least twice a week)
  B. Must take the formal Disciple Initiation Ceremony and Vow after the disciple test.

II. Crane Requirements
  A. Hsing   Competence in the performance of the:
   1. Wu Tai Hsing (Five Elements Form)
   2. Pai He Chuan (White Crane form)
   3. Wu Hsing Chuan (Five Animal Form)
  B. Chi Kung   Including the:
   1. energy visualizations in all hsing
   2. affirmations in all hsing
   3. All Mudra and Mudra meanings
   4. Understand and Explain the Five Animal symbolism

III. Snake Requiriments
  A. Uddiyana Pranayama (performed three times before Anuloma Viloma practice)
  B. Anuloma Viloma (performed before Crane Breath practice)
  C. Know the Chakra affirmations
  D. Know the Monk's Vow from memory

IV. Academic
  A. Presentation of one essay
    Subject: The Value of Passing on Tradition
  B. Presentation of one essay
    Subject: The Universality of Religion
  C. Read two books and submit a written paragraph
    on each of the 25 most important points in each book (Books are assigned by the director)

V. Character
  A. Integrity
  B. Has made self development an ultimate concern
  C. Has accepted a self disciplined life
  D. Has accepted responsibility for all of ones behaviors and all of ones circumstances.
  E. Has established a daily habit of consciousness energization, meditation and prayer

VI. Leadership
  A. Accept responsibility for the facilitation of holistic growth of self and all others
  B. Show competency in directing discipline in the Tao Chang

7 - 8   Monastic Requirements   Reading Requirements for Disciple Monk

Disciple Monk: Academic and Reading Requirements Description

Essay - Subject: <u>The Value of Passing on Tradition</u>

Purpose: At this level, one is accepting the responsibility of passing on the Shaolin Tradition. Correct motivation of this activity is essential. An understanding of what motivates our activities is also essential for efficient self development. As this essay is written it is hoped that the appropriateness of one's motivations are thoroughly examined and conclusions acted upon to further the process of personality purification and make you more fit to pass on the Shaolin Tradition.

Essay - Subject: <u>The Universality of Religion</u>

Purpose: The unfolding of spiritual awareness depends on an understanding that the Truth at the core of all the major religions of the world is the same. And, the different words used to refer to the One by the various languages and cultures of the world are just that; different words that refer to the same thing. Even within the Christian Tradition the different cultures and languages of the people contributing to the literature in the Bible used different words to refer to the One (ie. Elohim, Yaweh, God, Father, E'li, Adoni, Christ, Son of God, Lord, etc.). The people using these different words may have had slightly different aspects of the One in mind as these words were used, but these words are still referring to the One.

   The prospective Level Two student is to elaborate on this idea in this essay, incorporating concepts of the One from all the great religions of the world.

Read Two Books: director assigned books

   As each book is read, the testee will take notes on the most important points each book makes. The notes on the most important points made in each chapter will be submitted. Also, when the testee has finished reading each book, the 25 most important points the book makes will be selected. A paragraph explaining each of the 25 most important points will be submitted (25 paragraphs, one on each point), on each of the two books. In addition the testee **may** submit 25, four answer, multiple choice questions concerning each of the most important points, on each book. The testee will have the option of orally presenting the tests to a class.

Monastic Requirements — Requirements for Monk

I. General
   A. At least one year as a Disciple Monk, with regular class attendance
   B. Must take the formal Monk and Cobra Breath Initiation and Vow,

II. Crane Requirements
   A. Hsing
      Competence in the performance of the:
      1. San Zan Chuan (Monk Version)
      2. Sei San Chuan (Monk Version)
      3. San Sei Chuan (Monk version)
      4. Pai He No Kon
      5. Pai She Chuan
   B. Chi Kung   Including the:
      1. energy visualizations in all hsing
      2. affirmations in all hsing
      3. All Mudra and Mudra meanings in all hsing

III. Snake Requirements
   A. Maha Mudra with Chakra Mantra (practicing prior to test)
   B. Udiyana with Kustastha (practicing prior to test)
   C. Yoni Mudra with Kustastha (practicing prior to test)
   D. Cobra Breath (initiation and instruction before this test is administered)

IV. Academic
   A. Presentation of one research paper
      Subject: <u>Chi Kung</u>
   B. Presentation of second research paper
      Subject: <u>Yoga</u>
   C. Read five books and submit a written paragraph
      on each of the 25 most important points in each book (Books are assigned by the director)

V. Character
   A. Integrity
   B. Has made self development an ultimate concern
   C. Has accepted a self disciplined life
   D. Has accepted responsibility for all of ones behaviors and all of ones circumstances.
   E. Has established a daily habit of:
            consciousness energization, meditation, prayer and pranayama

VI. Leadership
   A. Accept responsibility for the facilitation of holistic growth of self and all others
   B. Show competency in directing discipline in the Tao Chang

Monk: Academic and Reading Requirements Description
Research Paper - Subject: Chi Kung

Purpose: The practice of Chi Kung holds the promise of enhancing one's health, vitality, youthfulness and longevity throughout the life time. At its most advanced levels of practice it is performed to bring spiritual insight and self-realization. It was taught within the Yogic Traditions of India as pranayama well into prehistoric times. At the very beginning of the Shaolin Tradition, Bodhidarma taught Chi Kung to the monks at the temple. As one recognized as qualified to pass on the teachings, a Level 3 student must have knowledge and direct experience of this integral and very important part of the Shaolin Tradition.

This research paper must demonstrate a knowledge of theory and practice of Chi Kung. Concepts to be covered are Jieng, Chi, Shen, Yi, Hsin, Kan, Lii and how these concepts are used to enhance the practice of Chi Kung. Wai Dan and Nei Dan theory and practice must be explained. Regulation of the body, breath, mind, essence, chi, and spirit in the application of Chi Kung must be explained. The use of the energy centers, vessels, channels and cavities in the practice of Chi Kung must be demonstrated in the paper. Recommendations for practice, detrimental side effects and remedies must be listed.

Research paper - Subject: Yoga

Purpose: One who has chosen this "way" and has come this far has made a commitment to total and complete personal development (perfection of the physical, mental and spiritual aspects of the self). This was and is the goal of the Shaolin Tradition. The monks and priests of this tradition looked to any source of information or discipline that would assist them in this endeavor. The most used source came from the Yogic Traditions of India. Through the centuries yogis from India were accepted in China and the Shaolin Temple many times, to teach their methods of holistic personal development. To make the most efficient progress toward this goal the Shaolin Monk should have this information.

This research paper must show an understanding of the laws of Yama and Niyama, karma, physical purification techniques, asana, mudra, banda, pranayama, pratyahara, dharana, meditation, mantra, samadhi.

Read Five Books: director assigned books

As each book is read, the testee will take notes on the most important points each book makes. The notes on the most important points made in each chapter will be submitted. Also, when the testee has finished reading each book, the 25 most important points the book makes will be selected. A paragraph explaining each of the 25 most important points will be submitted (25 paragraphs, one on each point), on each of the two books. In addition the testee **may** submit 25, four answer, multiple choice questions concerning each of the most important points, on each book. The testee will have the option of orally presenting the tests to a class.

Monastic Requirements

COBRA BREATH WARNING - Monk Requirements

The Cobra Breath and Warning

The Cobra Breath is an advanced consciousness energization method that will also perform personality purification functions. With sincere disciplined effort, Cobra Breath Training will put jet engines behind meditation ability. Instruction in the cobra breath requires preparatory training, vows and initiation from a Priest.

It is imperative that one is prepared before one begins Cobra Breath Training; Love, Compassion and Self Discipline *must* be sufficiently developed. Without the adequate levels of Love and Compassion, the motivation will not be strong enough to remain steadfast on the Path, let alone to sustain the required discipline and effort to accomplish the goal.

1) As a result of the Cobra Breath Training, mental abilities are significantly enhanced and if not used appropriately will cause suffering for the self and others. With enhanced mental abilities the potential for inappropriate behavior also grows. The karmic debt will grow proportionately to any inappropriateness. The suffering and the set back that will result can be staggering.

2) Sexual energy levels are dramatically raised so it is required that the motivation is pure and that the self discipline is developed enough to control energy loss. The high-energy levels and vitality are required for health and longevity. If adequate control is not attained: the sexual addiction will become stronger and even harder to overcome (eventually it *must* be over come), the energy levels will deflate causing immune system degeneration; the health will deteriorate, and the physical transition will come early.

Without the purification of consciousness and adequate control of energy loss,
the energization of consciousness will not occur.
The goal will not be achieved for many more lifetimes.
With this knowledge and these vows come responsibility.
When this responsibility is not met; more karmic debt.

Application for cobra breath initiation can be made to the director of the Shaolin Temple.
An application form can be found in the appendix A - 2.
The monk readiness assessment can be found in the appendix A - 3, A - 4, A - 5.
The address can be found in the appendix D - 1.

"Know ye not that ye are the temple of God, and that the spirit of God dwelleth in you?
For the temple of God is holy, which temple ye are." - I. Corinthians 3.16-17

7 - 12   **Monastic Requirements**   Requirements for Priest

I. General
   A. At least one year as a Monk, with regular class attendance
   B. Age - must be at least Thirty years old
   C. Must take the formal Initiation Ceremony and Vow of Priesthood

II. Crane Requirements
   A. Hsing
      Competence in the performance of all monk forms. Including the:
      1. energy visualizations
      2. affirmations
      3. All Mudra and Mudra meanings
   B. Chi Kung
      1. The energy accumulation techniques used in the performance of the hsing

III. Snake Requiriments
   A. Energy center opening yoga sequence
      1. Explaining visualizations
      2. Demonstrating postures
      3. Incorporating affirmations
   B. Cobra Breath with multiple upper chakra mantra reps
   C. Cobra Breath w/108 repetitions, daily

IV. Academic
   A. Presentation of one essay
      Subject: The Responsibilities of a Priest
   B. Presentation of one research paper
      Subject: The Why, When, Where, and How of Ceremony Performance
   C. Presentation of second research paper
      Subject: Methods used for Psychic Healing
   D. Read ten books and submit a written paragraph
      on each of the 25 most important points in each book (Books are assigned by the director)

V. Character
   A. Integrity
   B. Has made self development an ultimate concern
   C. Has accepted the self disciplined life of a Shaolin
   D. Has accepted responsibility for all of ones behaviors and all of ones circumstances.
   E. Has established a daily habit of: consciousness energization, meditation and prayer

VI. Leadership
   A. Accept responsibility for the facilitation of holistic growth of self and all others
   B. Show competency in directing discipline in the Tao Chang
   C. Show ability to run a Tao Chang
   D. Teaches own class at least weekly

Priest: Academic and Reading Requirements Description

Essay - Subject: <u>The Responsibilities of a Priest</u>

Purpose: The responsibilities to the self and others are common knowledge to a seeker of truth on any path. A Priest must have knowledge of responsibility to the Greater Self. In this essay the prospective Priest must explain this responsibility.

Research Paper - Subject: <u>The Why, When, Where, and How of Ceremony Performance</u>

Purpose: The purpose is to develop your ability to perform ceremonies and rituals. Some Ceremonies to cover are: Purification, Marriage, Baptism, Funeral, Rites of Passage, Transformative Rituals, etc.

Research Paper - Subject: <u>Methods used for Psychic Healing</u>

Purpose: Psychic healing techniques have been used by people of all cultures from the beginning of our time. The monks and priests at the Shaolin Temple were no exception. They were and are very adept in the use of these techniques. A Priest practicing within this tradition must have knowledge of these healing methods. This research paper must exhibit an understanding of these types of healing techniques. Examples of these techniques are prayer, visualization, reiki, Chi Kung, Pranayama, hypnosis, exorcism.

Read Ten Books: director assigned books

As each book is read, the testee will take notes on the most important points each book makes. The notes on the most important points made in each chapter will be submitted. Also, when the testee has finished reading each book, the 25 most important points the book makes will be selected. A paragraph explaining each of the 25 points will be submitted (25 paragraphs, one on each point), on each of the two books. In addition the testee **may** submit 25, four answer, multiple choice questions concerning each of the most important points, on each book. The testee will have the option of orally presenting the tests to a class.

APPENDIX

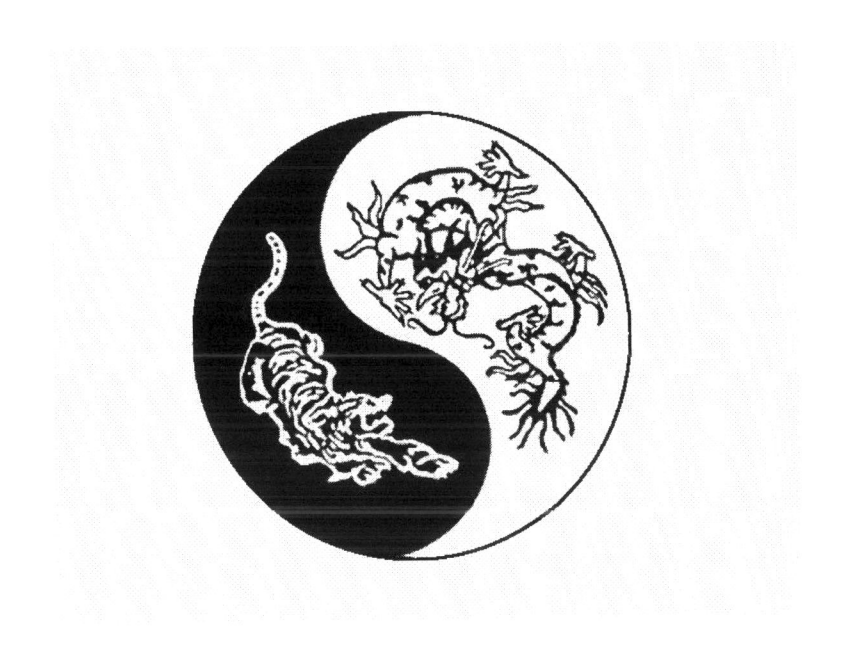

Appendix A **Self Analysis Chart** A - 1

This assessment is to be used privately, as each test is passed.
Identify your strong and weak points by marking yourself on each of the qualities listed below, marking yourself form 1 to 7 using the following scale:

Nearly Perfect	1	Above Average	3	Below Average	5	Almost Wholly Lacking	7
Good	2	Average	4	Deficient	6		

Avoid extremes of either pessimism or optimism. The more accurate you are the more meaning this will have.

Physical Qualities

__ physical vitality
__ general health
__ pleasing facial expression
__ personal neatness
__ appropriate dress
__ bodily control
　　nervous mannerisms
__ habits of hygiene
__ flexibility
__ speed
__ timing
__ agility
__ balance
__ strength
__ stamina
__ precision of movement
__ coordination
__ breath control
__ effective use of time

Mental Qualities

__ concentration
__ imagination
__ perseverance
__ memory
__ creativity
__ discipline
__ discrimination
__ objectivity
__ attention to detail
__ punctuality
__ verbal ability
__ sound judgement
__ self control
__ ability to develop self
__ knowledge
__ poise
__ courtesy
__ stability
__ helpfulness
__ tact
__ initiative
__ industry
__ resourcefulness
__ organization skill
__ spiritual awareness

Spiritual Qualities

__ intuition
__ humility
__ devotion
__ will
__ joyful
__ peaceful
__ wisdom
__ patience
__ courage
__ sincerity
__ trustworthiness
__ energy
__ stability
__ self confidence
__ gentleness
__ acceptance of others
__ love for all
__ compassion
__ charity
__ morality, personal habits
__ concern for
　　personal development
__ willingness to
　　accept suggestions
__ Ability to accept criticism

What five qualities are you most happy within yourself?

Look over your responses and note five qualities you are most concerned with improving.

Describe two ways you can work to develop each of these.

A - 2   **Appendix** (continued)
Application for Monk Level Advancement and/or Initiation

Name _____ Date _____
Address _____ Tele _____

City/State/Zip _____

With the submission of this application I agree to abide by all policies and rules of the Shaolin Temple, and to use my vow and training to further the holistic growth of myself and others. Furthermore, I agree to abide by the Vow of the Shaolin Monk. I realize that failure to comply with this vow may result in immediate and permanent dismissal from this association.

Signature of applicant _____

On this application please explain the what and why of this request and what has been done to qualify.

_____
_____
_____
_____
_____
_____
_____
_____
_____

This initiation application must be submitted:
1) at least one week prior to the selected date
2) with all written requirements   (ex. Monk Readiness, Self Assessment, Book Reports)
3) donation.

Monk Readiness
Self Assessment
A Sacred Practice

Introduction

The Shaolin Temple Monk Program is designed to provide a path for those individuals seeking to develop spiritual awareness through holistic personal growth and improving the quality of their life. This program focuses on having a healthy body and mind which assists in the development of spiritual awareness (developing a complete understanding and experience of Love, Wisdom and Truth).

This path is for those who recognize that life is a classroom where lesson after lesson is presented to us until we learn from each one in the process of perfection. Efficient progress in the development of these life lessons demands active and persistent pursuit. As one develops they will be able to have access to higher energy levels, heightened awareness, developed mental capacities and self defense abilities. As development continues and maturity occurs, there is a positive influence on those around us as well as all of humanity.

Joining the Shaolin Monk Program, is a decision that is to be taken seriously. It requires a commitment of time, patience and dedication to learn and integrate the principles and teachings of the Shaolin Temple into one's life.

The methods used in personal and spiritual development have been passed down to us by generations of highly advanced monks for literally thousands of years. They are compatible with the practices of all the great religions of the world.

By responding truthfully as you go through the Assessment of Readiness, you will be matched with the preparations necessary for you to be initiated into the Shaolin Monk Program.

We look forward to sharing this journey with you.

With Love, Light and Joy.
The Monks of Shaolin

A - 4   **Appendix** (continued)   **Monk Readiness, Self-Assessment** (continued)

Directions: Using a separate piece of paper, please respond to the following questions. When finished, please return this question sheet along with your responses to the Shaolin Temple.

Please **Print** or **Type** your responses.

1. What motivated you to apply to the monk program?

2. List the books related to personal and/or spiritual development that you have read in the last three years.

3. Who was the founder of the Shaolin tradition and what was his relevant background?

4. What are the goals of the Shaolin Tradition?

5. Explain the four requirements within the Shaolin Method of personal growth.

6. Define *Purification of personality* and *Energization of consciousness* and explain how they are different.

7. Define and explain, sthana and samasthana, and use your sthana as an example in your explanation.

8. Explain the four stages and the goal of meditation?

9. How often do you meditate and why?

Monk Readiness, Self-Assessment (continued)   **Appendix** (continued)   A - 5

10. Describe the chakra morality orientation construct and using this construct assess your moral development using examples of your thoughts and behaviors.

11. Name and describe the Five Perfections of the Shaolin Tradition.

12. What purpose do the Five Perfections serve? Explain how you will use the Five Perfections to accomplish this purpose.

13. Define mudra and explain the purpose of mudra performance.

14. What is the purpose of form performance?

15. Define spiritual ignorance and explain its impact on the individual and on humanity.

16. Is it important to develop your intuition? Explain your answer.

17. Explain your understanding of Self Examination and why Self Examination is important. In your explanation include the use of ego defense mechanisms and list the ego defense mechanisms that you are using.

18. Explain your understanding of the Crane Breath and the Cobra Breath and the importance of each.

Tao Chang Rules

Tao Chang Rules

1. Know that the Tao Chang is a place that is due great respect, since it is a place where people come to further their personal growth.
2. Everyone must be courteous, respectful and helpful to others at all times.
3. Senior students are responsible for enforcing the Tao Chang rules. Senior students must act in an exemplary manner.
4. <u>Students</u> must maintain a clean and orderly Tao Chang.
5. Horseplay and loud talking are forbidden.
6. Kicking and punching the Tao Chang walls are forbidden.
7. Eating, drinking and gum chewing in the training area are forbidden.
8. Shoes are to be removed at the door and set out of the doorway in or under the shoe-rack.
9. Everyone must remain fully dressed in the Tao Chang.
10. Only the Tao Chang patch may be worn on the uniform.
11. Student should be on time for the class they are to participate in.
12. Students are responsible for stretching out and warming up before class begins.
13. While class is in progress no one will leave the line-up except for emergencies such as illness, exhaustion, etc.
14. During the class opening and closing ceremonies, every student present will participate.
15. Students entering and leaving the class must walk around the line-up.
16. Student's bodies and uniforms must be kept clean. Pungent body odor is indicative of a lack of respect for self and others. Strong perfumes and aftershaves are not to be used.
17. No one is ever to do anything that could be dangerous to one's self or anyone else.
18. It is necessary that everyone use a complete set of adequate protectors to avoid injury during partner practice.
19. Wearing jewelry while class is in progress is forbidden.
20. Weapons practice is allowed only after regular classes.
21. All students must keep finger nails and toe nails trimmed short to prevent injury to themselves and others.
22. Students should pay constant attention to what is being taught and put as much effort as possible into what is being attempted.
23. Unnecessary talking during class is forbidden. Comments, and most questions, should be delayed until after class.
24. Students must know that Koei Kan Ken Do Gaku was originated as a study. Its goal is for its practitioners to obtain the highest level of human maturity possible through the study. To achieve this end, practitioners must overcome many difficulties to realize their greater self. Practitioners must become strong enough to rely on their own good judgement and develop the discipline required so as to not get lost in the ways of the world or one's own selfishness.

Bibliography B - 1

Suggested Reading List   Required Reading *

An Easy Guide to Ayurveda: Roy Eugene Davis
1996, CSA Press   ISBN 0-87707-249-3

Ageless Body, Timeless Mind: Deepak Chopra
1993, Harmony Books   ISBN 0-517-59257-6

* The Art of Loving: Erick Fromm
1974, Perennial Library

* Autobiography of a Yogi: Paramahansa Yogananda
1993, Self Realization Fellowship   ISBN 0-87612-079-6

The Bhagavad Gita: translated by Paramahansa Yogananda
1995, Self Realization Fellowship   ISBN 0-87612-030-3

* Change your Thoughts - Change your Life, Living the Wisdom of the Tao:
Dr. Wayne W. Dyer 2007, Hay House, Inc. ISBN: 978-1-4019-1184-3

*The Bodhisattva Warriors: Shifu Nagaboshi Tomio (Terence Dukes)
1994, Samuel Weiser, Inc.   ISBN 0-87728-785-6

* The Eternal Way: Roy Eugene Davis
1996, CSA Press   ISBN 0-87707-248-5

Gifts from Eykis: Dr. Wayne Dyer
1984, Pocket Books   ISBN 0-671-68461-2

The Holy Bible: King James Version
Thomas Nelson Inc.

Jeet Kune Do Bruce Lee's Commentaries on the Martial Way:
Compiled and Edited by John Little
1997 Linda Lee Caldwell, Tuttle Publishing ISBN: 978-0-8048-3132-1

Life Surrendered in God: Roy Eugene Davis
1990, CSA Press   ISBN 0-87707-246-9

Man's Eternal Quest: Paramahansa Yogananda
1982, Self-Realization Fellowship   ISBN 0-87612-232-2

Bibliography (continued)

* A Master Guide to Meditation: Roy Eugene Davis
1994, CSA Press   ISBN 0-87707-238-8

The Path of Light: Roy Eugene Davis
1998, CAS Press   ISBN 0-87707-277-9

* A New Earth, Awakening to Your Life's Purpose: Eckhart Tolle
2005, Plume   ISBN 978-0-452-28996-3

* Reinventing the Body, Resurrecting the Soul: Deepak Chopra
Three Rivers Press   ISBN 978-0-307-45298-6

The Road Less Traveled: M. Scott Peck, M.D.
1978, Simon & Schuster   ISBN 0-671-25067-1

The Root of Chinese Chi Kung: Dr. Yang Jwing-Ming
1989, Yang's Martial Arts Association   ISBN 0-940871-07-6

The Sacred Pipe: Black Elk   recorded and edited by Joseph Epes Brown
1953, 1989, University of Oklahoma Press, ISBN 0-8061-2124-6

* The Science of Self Realization   The Yoga Sutras and Commentary   Roy Davis
2000, CSA Press

The Second Coming of Christ - The Resurrection of Christ Within You:
Paramahansa Yogananda
2004, Self Realization Fellowship   ISBN 0-87612-555-0

The Self-Revealed Knowledge that Liberates the Spirit: Roy Eugene Davis
1997, CSA Press   ISBN 0-87707-275-2

Seven Lessons in Conscious Living: Roy Eugene Davis
2000, CSA Press   ISBN 0-87707-280-9

The Seven Spiritual Laws of Success: Deepak Chopra
1993, Amber-Allen Publishing   ISBN 1-878424-11-4

Bibliography (continued)

The Tao-Teh-King sayings of Lao Tzu: translated C. Spurgeon Medhurst
1975, The Theosophical Publishing House   ISBN: 0-8356-0430-6

Transformative Rituals: Gay and David Williamson
1994, Health Communications, Inc.   ISBN 1-55874-293-X

Your Erroneous Zones: Dr. Wayne W. Dyer
1977, Avon Books   ISBN 0-380-01669-9

The Way of Herbs: Michael Tierra
1980, Washington Square Press   ISBN 0-671-46686-0

The Way of the Wizard: Deepak Chopra
1995, Harmony Books   ISBN 0-517-70434-X

Wicca: Scott Cunningham
1997, Llewellyn Publications   ISBN 0-87542-118-0

* The Zen Teachings of Bodhidaharma: Translated by Red Pine
1987, 1) Empty Bowl 2) North Point Press   ISBN 0 86547 399 4

Glossary of Terms

attachment - attachments are your possessions, thoughts and deeds that you believe are required for you to experience security, happiness and Joy. At the root of attachments are false perceptions that will tie you to the material realm and prevent you from having a direct experience of Spirit. Attachments are creations of the ego that it uses to try to get by in the world. Since the ego's perception of reality is **very** limited, its conclusions and decisions are usually inappropriate. Attachments are no exception. So when it discovers that an attachment is no longer working (very often with considerable stress and often suffering) it will drop that attachment and find another. This is a repeating cycle. It can, and most often does, happen over and over again for many, many lifetimes. The cycle will not end until the ego's perception of reality matures with a direct experience of Spirit.

ayurveda (Sanskrit term) - is a several thousand year old system of holistic health maintenance and medical therapy with origins in India. The system uses diet, herbs, water therapy, massage, attitude training, detoxification regimens, meditation, etc. to restore and maintain a condition of energy balance in the body.

believe - to know (note; you **can not** know or believe something just because you have been told or read about it). Most things written or spoken about are not true due to limited knowledge or intentional deception. Belief and knowledge require direct experience. See *worldly paradigm*.

bhujang pranayama (Sanskrit term) - cobra breath. (See *cobra breath*)

Bodhisattva (Sanskrit term) - one who knows that real liberation can not occur without the liberation of all beings, since all beings are part of the Supreme Unity. Due to Perfect Compassion, the Bodhisattva will forgo complete union with Spirit to help unenlightened beings overcome suffering through the development of spiritual awareness. Even after dharma-megha samadhi, the Bodhisattva will remain within creation assisting unenlightened sentient beings until all become enlightened. Sanskrit term.

bogu (Japanese term) - A term for protective equipment worn during fighting practice

bu (Chinese term) - The term for stance. Some examples of stances are:
Wan Bu - the bow stance
Ma Bu - horse stance
He Bu - crane stance
She Bu - snake stance
Long Bu - dragon stance
Bao Bu - panther stance
Mao Bu - cat stance
Vajra Bu - lightning bolt stance, San Zan stance
Ssu Lieu Bu - reverse bow stance, back stance
Dsao Pan Bu - cross leg stance
Hu Bu - tiger stance
Tian Di Bu - heaven and earth stance

Buddha (Sanskrit term) - 1) One who has attained complete and perfect Enlightenment. 2) Siddhartha Gautama (563-483 B.C.) Known as the Buddha, founder of Buddhism (also known as the Universal Religion). He taught the Yogic ideals in what he called The Eight Fold Path and The Five Commands of Uprightness with an emphasis on non-violence.

Glossary of Terms (continued)

Brahma (Sanskrit term) - 1) The principle of creation. 2) One of the Hindu Trinity (Brahma, Vishnu and Shiva).

Chan or Chan'na (Chinese term) - Buddhist sect founded by Bodhidarma circa 525 AD. Chan'na is the Chinese rendering of the Sanskrit term dhyana and means meditation. Meditation is the primary method used in Chan Buddhism for developing Spiritual Awareness. This is based on the concept that at their core, all beings are Spirit and that meditation is used to allow the consciousness to experience its core. This experience will bring the awareness of what we actually are, Spirit. The Japanese refer to Chan Buddhism as *Zen*.

chi (Chinese term) - A term for the energy created by Spirit and used to manifest creation and everything in it. Sometimes called *internal energy*. The Sanskrit term is *prana*. (page 4 - 1)

chi kung (Chinese term) - methods of internal energy (chi) control, used for: 1) energy accumulation, conservation, transportation of chi 2) health maintenance 3) developing spiritual awareness. In the yogic tradition, chi kung is known as *pranayama*.
There are two types of chi kung: 1) Wai Dan Chi Kung. Wai Dan Chi Kung, are the methods used to accumulate chi in localized areas of the body. 2) Nei Dan Chi Kung. Nei Dan Chi Kung is used to accumulate and transport chi through the chi vessels and meridians of the body. The chi vessels and meridians make up the chi circulatory system. Chi balancing and distribution can assist in controlling health, vitality, longevity, mental acuity and spiritual awareness.

class ceremonies - (see page 7 - 5)

Cobra Breath - is an advanced consciousness energization method that will also perform personality purification functions. Instruction in the cobra breath requires previous training, vows and initiation.

concentration - The ability to focus the mind on what ever is being attended to; eliminating extraneous thought. (See dharana)

consciousness - six levels
    unconscious, deep sleep
    subconscious, dream states
    ego conscious, ordinary waking state
    Super conscious, awareness of ones soul and soul memories
    Christ conscious, awareness of Spirit within creation
    Cosmic conscious, awareness of Spirit beyond creation

courage - The ability to take a risk even in the face of disappointment and pain, to behave according to values that are personally judged to be of supreme importance.

Glossary of Terms (continued)　　　C - 3

dan (Japanese term) - A term for Black Belt level, literally "mature person".
One becomes mature when the individual can operate psychologically, unaffected by influences outside the self. From the spiritual perspective, one becomes mature when one has had an experience of enlightenment.

dharana (Sanskrit term) - the ability to hold thought on one concept for an extended period of time. This ability is required for efficient meditation. In meditation, the concept used is an aspect of The Great Spirit (Love, Light, Wisdom, Joy etc.).

dharma (Sanskrit term) - path to Spirit. Behaviors and thoughts one uses to obtain Self and God Realization. The "law" of Spirit, Truth; All knowledge and Wisdom. Second in the Triratna: 1)Buddha 2) Dharma 3) Sangha. Sangha is the spiritual community or the Order of Monks.

detachment - to expose and release attachments, false perceptions and all delusion from the consciousness (this is required for efficient development of spiritual awareness).
The antonym is attachment; which is to identify yourself with your possessions, thoughts and deeds and believe that your possessions, thoughts and deeds are required for you to experience security and happiness. Attachment will tie you to the material realm and prevent you from having a direct experience of Spirit.

dhyana (Sanskrit term) - word for meditation. Concentration used to experience Spirit.

discipline - The ability to stick it out and pursue the correct behavior (e.g. exercise, kindness, etc.) even when not in the mood.

dojo (Japanese term) - A term for a place where martial arts are practiced for the development of spiritual wisdom. *Tao Chang* in Chinese. *Bodhimandala* in Sanskit.

ego - 1) A usually unconscious aspect of the personality and belief system, that the personality creates to interact with its physical and social environment. It is most often based on inappropriate conclusions and creates an inaccurate perception of reality (the *worldly paradigm*). It is the cause of all stress and suffering. 2) The delusive awareness of individuality.

enlightenment - The experience of the dissolution of the ego. This occurs when the intuition apprehends the unity of humanity, life, creation and Spirit. The awareness experiences its self as part of Spirit and all of the aspects of Spirit as its self; including Infinite Divine Love. This is the accurate apprehension of Reality and results in a total release from stress and suffering.

faith - is belief that your own ability to reason and intuit will eventually bring complete Spiritual realization and using information gained from your abilities to come to your own conclusions and behave accordingly in spite of the majority's opinion, social pressure or any extrinsic influence.

Glossary of Terms (continued)

form - a ritual movement involving the performance of a prearranged sequence of movement; usually including mudra and or martial technique. It is a method of self examination, personality purification and physical exercise. It can be used as a physical preparation for spiritual chi kung and can include spiritual chi kung methods. The Chinese word for form is *hsing*, Japanese is *kata* and Sanskrit is *nata*.

God - The infinite, omnipresent, omniscient, omnipotent consciousness that pervades the universes and beyond. It is infinite: Love, Wisdom, Joy, Peace and Bliss. The Great Spirit.

Grade and Monastic Level   1) Student Monk   2) Disciple Monk   3) Monk   4) Priest

intuition - the "sixth sense", the ability, when developed, that enables one to gain infallible knowledge and /or insight directly from the soul.

hsing (Chinese term) - A Chinese term for the English word *form*. See *form*.

hsiu hsing (Chinese term) - Any training method, practice, or rite used to purify the personality. Its use is etymologically related to the Sanskrit word *kriya* and the Japanese word *shugyo*.

karma (Sanskrit term) - the natural law of cause and effect at the spiritual level. It is the reaction of the universe to one's thoughts and deeds to achieve balance. Each person's thoughts and actions determine what is experienced; good thoughts and behavior will attract more good. Thoughts and behavior that cause suffering to oneself or to others will cause more suffering. This Cosmic Law is the motivator of immature personalities to positive change, and ultimately to enlightenment .

kata (Japanese term) - A term for the English word *form*. See *form*.

kihon (Japanese term) - A term for martial technique practice (i.e. punches, kicks, blocks)

kiai (Japanese term) - A term for a loud shout used to focus *kime* into a maximum physical effort.

kime (Japanese term) - A term for an application of complete mental concentration.

klesa (Sanskrit term) - Bodhidharma spoke of the Klesa as psychological poison and inner demons. According to Bodhidharma, these inner demons are the three causes of human suffering: 1) self centeredness, (greed, attachments, etc.) 2) ignorance* 3) fear (hatred etc.). *Ignorance would include all delusion (erroneous mental concepts and ideas) and illusion (misperception of facts); also the act of ignoring Truth and Wisdom. Basic ego awareness and confusion would be considered ignorance. These are concepts used in the personality purification process of self examination required for the development of spiritual awareness. See also the *worldly paradigm*.

Glossary of Terms (continued)

Gnostics - Probably the earliest sect of Christianity. It was to this sect that the mystic teachings of Jesus were taught; definitely predating the constantinian influence.

kriya (Sanskrit term) - an ancient science developed in India that will lead seekers to experience cosmic consciousness. This includes pranayama methods and chi kung methods taught and practiced at the Shaolin Temple. Historically related to the Chinese term *hsiu hsing* and the Japanese term *shugyo* which mean *let us prepare for enlightenment.*

lohan (Chinese term) - A bodhisattva monk who has made a solemn vow to do everything possible to achieve buddhahood (self-realization and God-realization) within the present incarnation.

mantra (Sanskrit term) - syllables, words and or phrases representing spiritual concepts and used to focus the mind for meditation and expand spiritual awareness.

meditation - concentration used to know and experience God.

mystic - A seeker who believes that one can apprehend and experience knowledge, Wisdom and the Ultimate Reality by looking into the self with the use of intuition. Meditation is the tool most commonly used to facilitate this ability and experience.

objectivity - The ability to think logically, to use pertinent data in thought processes (e.i. decision making) eliminating rationalization, projection, repression, denial, transference, etc.

patience - Good natured tolerance for delay. Required for the development of spiritual awareness.

pranayama (Sanskrit term) - breath control and visualizations used to energize the consciousness. These are consciousness energization exercises required to raise intuition levels high enough to experience Spirit. Examples are the crane breath and the cobra breath.

pratyahara (Sanskrit term) - withdrawal of mental attention from sense sensations (auditory, visual, olfactory, tactile) to enhance concentration during meditation.

rishi (Sanskrit term) - an enlightened seer

root - achieving a sense of strong stability in ones stance and posture. This can be used as a foundation for launching powerful martial technique and to enhance some methods of chi kung.

salvation - christian term for union with God.

samadhi (Sanskrit term) - a yogic term, unbroken focused attention that results in the personal experience of union with God. Also see *enlightenment*.

Glossary of Terms (continued)

samasthana (Sanskrit term) - The process of self examination - personality purification. (See page 2 - 2)

sanshou (Chinese term) - Formal martial training match, performed with the primary goal of holistic development of all those involved. An emphasis on personal detachment and samasthana are administered during the performance of this activity. (See page 2 - 11)

satori (Japanese term) - Zen Buddhist term, for the personal experience of union with God.

self - There are three basic levels of self perception and self awareness.
    1) ego awareness - this is the level of awareness that most people operate within. (see ego)
    2) soul awareness - aware that one is an immortal spiritual being. (see soul)
    3) Spirit awareness - fully aware that the Great Spirit is the source of one's being. (see Spirit)

self disciplined life - living a life: 1) eliminating all vices and unhealthy habits 2) adopting habits and practices conducive to positive personal growth.

sensei (Japanese term) - term for teacher; in the Shaolin Kung Fu Martial Arts Association, teacher level is Level Three or above and has completed the Teacher Certification Requirements.

sentient being - are beings that have the power of perception through their senses.

siddha (Sanskrit term) - an enlightened being, a "perfected" person, a yoga master.

shiai (Japanese term) - A term for non-competitive, spontaneous give and take fighting practice with detachment and *samasthana*, for learning and promotional analysis. Chinese term is *san shou*.

sifu or **shifu** (Chinese term) - A term for teacher.

single eye - the ajna chakra, this is the organ of intuition in humanity. The white star in the center is a portal into Spirit. See *Upper Tan Tien*

soul - an individualized unit of God - Spirit.

spinal centers - psychic energy centers along the spine that influence personality orientation and vitality levels. The 7 major chakra are: *muladhara, swadhisthana, manipura, anahata, vishudha, ajna, sahasrara*. (Sanskrit terms) (See page 4 - 4)

Spirit / God. - The infinite, omnipresent, omniscient, omnipotent consciousness that pervades the universes and beyond. Some of its aspects are infinite: Love, Wisdom, Joy, Peace and Bliss.

sthana (Sanskrit term) - A term for ego. (see *ego*)

Glossary of Terms (continued)

tao chang (Chinese term) - A term for a place where martial arts are practiced for the development of spiritual wisdom and enlightenment. Sanskrit term *bodhimandala*. Japanese term *dojo*.

taolu (Chinese term) - A term for martial technique practice (i.e. punches, kicks, blocks)

tenshin - A Japanese term that refers to 1) physical mobility 2) rotation of the body used to increase the efficiency of movement and develop power 3) adaptation to changing circumstances.

triratna (Sanskrit term) - the Three Jewels of Buddhism: The 1) *Buddha*, 2) *Dharma* (His Teachings), and the 3) *Sangha* (spiritual community or order of monks).

Truth - Truth is an aspect of Spirit, pertaining to or related to Reality.

ultimate concern - A direct experience of Spirit must be a matter of ultimate concern requiring intense active pursuit to make efficient progress.

ujjayi (Sanskrit term) - or sometimes spelt *ujaiya*. An inhale or exhale of the breath, constricting the throat to make the breath slightly audible. This breath is used in some *chi kung/pranayama* breathing methods.

Upper Tan Tien (Chinese term) - known variously as: the spiritual eye, the third eye, the Christ Consciousness center, the seat of the soul, the star of Bethlehem, ajna chakra, the Pentacle. This is the organ of intuition in humanity. It is located at the spot between the eye brows, in the area of the pituitary gland.

waza (Japanese term) - A term for martial technique practice, it can include partner practice.

worldly paradigm - is the faulty orientation to life created by the ego for the purpose of making sense out of reality and attempting to efficiently interact with it. The information the ego uses to develop this orientation is based on what it can get from the five senses and the minds ability to assemble the information into a usable form. The senses evolved to interact with the earth environment and nothing more, they can not collect information beyond creation. The problem is that the vast majority of Reality exits beyond creation, unaccessible to the senses and the intellect. Through the intellect alone, the ego does not have the knowledge or experience to apprehend Reality. The belief system based on this orientation is the cause of all stress and suffering. The only way to solve this problem is through a personal intuitive experience of Spirit.

wu hsin (Chinese term) - A state of mind that is free of thought (especially thought in word format) but totally aware. Used for meditation, the performance of forms and any spontaneous creative thought and /or action.

Glossary of Terms (continued)

yin and yang (Chinese term) - The polarity of internal energy that influences how matter and energy will behave (yin having a negative polarity and yang a positive). This is a Taoist concept probably originating from the Hindu concepts of Shiva and Vishnu (the influences that sustain the continued evolution within creation). See page 4-1

yoga (Sanskrit term) - A term for union with God (self-realization and God-realization) Refers to methods that bring together the body, mind and soul to achieve union with the infinite.

yudansha (Japanese term) - a black belt holder or an advanced grade level holder.

Zen (Sanskrit term) - This is Bodhidharma's term for self realization. Also, the Japanese use the term for the Shaolin Buddhist meditation sect Chan, established by Bodhidharma in 525 AD. The Zen Buddhist Sect was embraced by the Samurai Class of feudal Japan. The word *Zen* can refer: to *Satori*, to the meditation state, *wu-hsin*, or any thought or behavior that will bring more awareness of Spirit.

zhunbei (Chinese term) - a command usually used during a formal training class to call the students to attention and to stand at attention.

zhunbei bu (Chinese term) - ready stance, used to begin the performance of forms.

Instructional Aids

San Zan Chuan, Mudra and Chi Kung - DVD

Sei San Chuan - DVD

San Sei Chuan - DVD

Wu Shi Si - DVD

Bodhisattva Dao - DVD

Wu Hsing Chuan - The 5 Animal Form - DVD

Wu Tai Hsing - Form of the 5 Elements - DVD

Pai He Hsing - White Crane Hsing - DVD

Pai He No Kon - White Crane Staff - DVD

Yue Chia Hsing: Yi, Er, San, Si, Wu, - DVDs

Yang Kon Hsing - Staff - DVD

Lunar Spiritual Eye Energization Ritual - DVD

Audio CD
    Meditation - prayer and instructions
            with Singing Bowl
    San Zan Affirmation - at form speed
    Wu Tai Hsing Affirmation - at form speed
    Humanity Healing Ritual
            with Singing Bowl

Applications, DVDs and CDs are available from the:
Shaolin Temple of Michigan
6345 Newburgh Road
Westland, Michigan
48185

WWW.ShaolinTempleUS.org

Made in the USA
Columbia, SC
21 June 2024